Marina Viegas Moura R. Ribeiro

Efficacy of Platelet Concentrate in Diabetic Dry Eye

Marina Viegas Moura R. Ribeiro

Efficacy of Platelet Concentrate in Diabetic Dry Eye

Review and clinical case series

ScienciaScripts

Imprint

Cover image: www.ingimage.com

This book is a translation from the original published under ISBN 978-3-330-76677-8.

Publisher:
Sciencia Scripts
is a trademark of
Dodo Books Indian Ocean Ltd. and OmniScriptum S.R.L publishing group

120 High Road, East Finchley, London, N2 9ED, United Kingdom
Str. Armeneasca 28/1, office 1, Chisinau MD-2012, Republic of Moldova, Europe
Managing Directors: Ieva Konstantinova, Victoria Ursu
info@omniscriptum.com

Printed at: see last page
ISBN: 978-620-8-54451-5

I dedicate this work to my husband Luiz Eduardo Feliciano Ribeiro for his support and unconditional love.

ACKNOWLEDGEMENTS

To God for enlightening me to overcome obstacles;

To Prof. Dr Êurica Adélia Nueira Ribeiro Dr Êurica Adélia Nogueira Ribeiro for her trust, guidance and understanding;

To Prof Dr Fabiano Timbó Barbosa for his constant dedication, attention and collaboration;

To Prof Dr João Marcelo de Almeida Gusmão Lyra for his support;

To Prof. Dr Celina Maria Costa Lacet Dr Celina Maria Costa Lacet for her support and encouragement in preparing this work;

To Professor and Master Patrícia Costa Pinto, who allowed me to carry out my research, as well as to Professor and Director of the Alagoas Haemocentre (HEMOAL) Verônica Lima and her entire team;

To Dr Tadeu Cvintal, from the Tadeu Cvintal Ophthalmology Institute in São Paulo, for his ophthalmological knowledge, which I owe to him;

To Dr Nelson Tatsui, haematologist and director of Criogênesis, São Paulo, who first guided me through the preparation of the platelet concentrate;

To ophthalmologist and master Daniel Fridman, who provided me with teaching material and allowed me access to his dissertation;

To the faculty and students of the Postgraduate Programme in Health Sciences, who provided me with an ideal environment for my studies;

To my parents, Antônio Luiz and Marluce, for their affection and for making up for my absence from my children at important times; to my mother-in-law, Maria Cecília, for helping me to make progress in my home during this period; to my children, Maria Eduarda and Luiz Antônio, for being the meaning of my life; and to my husband, Luiz Eduardo, for all his support in revising and writing my dissertation;

And to everyone who contributed directly and indirectly to this stage of my life, thank you very much.

Co-Authors

Marina Viegas Moura Rezende Ribeiro - MSc in Health Sciences, Federal University of Alagoas, Brazil. Specialist in Ophthalmology. Adjunct Professor of Medicine at Tiradentes University.

Eurica Adélia Nogueira Ribeiro - PhD in Bioactive Natural and Synthetic Products, Federal University of Paraíba. Adjunct Professor Level I, Federal University of Alagoas, Brazil

Fabiano Timbó Barbosa - PhD in Health Sciences, Federal University of Alagoas, Brazil. Professor of the Postgraduate Programme in Health Sciences, Federal University of Alagoas.

Luiz Eduardo Feliciano Ribeiro - Specialist in Ophthalmology.

Patrícia Costa Alves Pinto. Master of Science, University of Health Sciences Alagoas. Specialist in paediatric haemotology.

SUMMARY

Diabetic dry eye has a very variable prevalence and its pathophysiology involves hyperglycaemia causing metabolic, neuropathic and vascular lesions. Conventional treatment with lubricants is often not enough in moderate to severe cases, which can lead to complications such as keratopathy, corneal opacities, eye perforations and loss of visual acuity. Platelet concentrate eye drops (POC) have already been used in ocular surface diseases due to their role in re-epithelialisation and the presence of growth factors and vitamins that resemble human tears. There are few studies reporting its use in dry eye, and none in diabetic dry eye. The main objective of this study was to evaluate the efficacy of CCP in symptomatic diabetic dry eye. To this end, a time-series clinical trial was carried out in which 12 diabetic patients refractory to conventional treatment used CCP for one month. The variables analysed before and after treatment were dry eye symptoms, clinical signs of the disease, visual acuity and objective Schirmer tests and tear film break-up time (TRFL), following the Dry Eye Workshop (DEWS) severity criteria, and the Ocular Surface Disease Index (OSDI). The patients improved in the following aspects: dry eye symptoms (p=0.002), 41.66 per cent in visual acuity (p=0.14), 66.67 per cent in the Schirmer test (p=0.04), 58.33 per cent in the TRFL (p=0.01), and 100 per cent in the OSDI score, with 56.13 ±20.94 before treatment, which corresponded to severe dry eye, and 13.15 ±11.40 after, leading to the absence of symptoms. We can therefore conclude that CCP is an effective alternative therapy for diabetic dry eye. However, more clinical trials are needed to create specific protocols and evaluate the effectiveness of this treatment.

Keywords: Dry eye. Diabetes. Platelet concentrate.

SUMMARY

CHAPTER 1

INTRODUCTION

1.1 Background

Diabetes can affect various organs, including the eyes, and can cause ocular complications such as diabetic retinopathy, cataracts, muscle paralysis with strabismus, myopia and also dry eye (MINISTÉRIO DA SÁUDE, 2006; PEREIRA; ARCHER; RUIZ, 2009). Diabetic dry eye can develop into changes in the ocular surface that can lead to irreversible complications such as severe keratopathy, with ocular perforation, trophic ulcers or corneal scarring (RIORDAN-EVA; WHITCHER, 2008).

According to recent consensus, dry eye or dry keratoconjunctivitis is a multifactorial disease of the tear and ocular surface that results in discomfort, visual disturbances and instability of the tear film, with potential risks of damage (DRY EYE WORKSHOP, 2007a). It affects between 5% and 34% of the general population, with women and the elderly being the groups most affected by this syndrome. The wide variation is due to variations in population studies, geographical variations, differences in the study method and differences in the definition of dry eye (MESSMER, 2015).

The prevalence of dry eye in diabetic patients ranges from 8.4 per cent in patients under 60 to 19 per cent in elderly patients (MOSS; KLEIN; KLEIN, 2004) and can reach 54.3 per cent in some studies (MANAVIAT et al., 2008). The pathophysiology involves metabolic, neuropathic and vascular lesions that lead to an inflammatory process and functional degeneration caused by hyperglycaemia, accumulation of advanced glycosylation end products, oxidative stress and inflammation (ALVES et al., 2008).

Dry eye presents two challenges: the controversial diagnosis, since the symptoms generally have no clinical correlation with existing objective tests, and the usual treatment, mainly with ocular lubricants that may not be effective in more severe cases (RAHMAN et al., 2007; LIU et al., 2005).

In the 1980s, with the aim of researching a treatment for dry eye that had properties closer to human tears, Fox et al. reported the benefits of autologous serum in patients with dry eye in Sjogren's syndrome. However, this was only put into practice when Tsubota et al demonstrated the efficacy of this therapy in a study of 12 dry eye patients at the end of the decade (FOX et al., 1984; TSUBOTA et al., 1999a).

Human serum or plasma is rich in epidermal growth factor, vitamin A, beta growth factor, fibronectin and cytokines that are found in tears, and bactericidal factors (immunoglobulins IgG and

IgA and lysozyme) that help keep the ocular surface healthy (KOFFLER, 2006). It has been advocated in various ophthalmological pathologies, in addition to dry eye, such as epithelial defects (TSUBOTA et al., 1999b; YOUNG et al., 2004; ALVARADO VALERO et al., 2004), corneal erosions, 2004), recurrent corneal erosions (DEL CASTILLO et al., 2002; HOLZER et al., 2005; REIDY; PAULUS; GONA, 2000), neurotrophic keratopathy (MATSUMOTO et al., 2004), trabeculectomy ampullae (MATSUO et al., 2005), superior limbic keratoconjunctivitis (GOTO et al., 2001), graft versus host disease (MIXON et al., 2014), post refractive surgery (NODA-TSURUYA et al., 2006), ocular surface reconstruction (TSUBOTA et al., 1996), Mooren's ulcer (MAVRAKANAS; KIEL; DOSSO, 2007) and aniridia keratopathy (LÓPEZ-GARCÍA et al., 2008).

However, it has been observed that platelet concentrate eye drops (POC) have higher levels of EGF (epithelial growth factor) and vitamin A than autologous serum, with rare reports of complications. Autologous serum also contains pro-inflammatory cytokines derived from leukocytes and monocytes, which in patients with immunological alterations or diseases can be deleterious; hence the advantage of platelet concentrate, as it is free of these inflammatory immunoglobulins (LIU et al., 2006; LÓPEZ-GARCÍA et al., 2014).

The use of CCP in ophthalmology for ocular surface diseases has been reported, as has autologous serum (KIM; SHIN; KIM, 2012; REZENDE et al., 2007; ALIO et al., 2007b; PANDA et al, 2012; MARQUEZ DE ARACENA DEL CID; MONTERO DE ESPINOSA ESCORIAZA, 2009; JAVALOY et al., 2013), in restoring tear function (MY, 2014), in blepharoplasties (VICK et al., 2006), among others.

Recently, its use in patients with dry eye of various causes has been reported by Lopez-Plandolit et al. and Alio et al. In the first study, which was carried out with 16 patients with dry eye refractory to the usual treatment, it was observed that 75% of the patients obtained an improvement in their condition without needing to use any other treatment. The second study assessed 18 patients who used CCP and of these 89% had an improvement in symptoms, 86% an improvement in conjunctival hyperaemia and 72% a significant improvement in keratitis (ALIO et al., 2007a; LÓPEZ-PLANDOLIT et al., 2011). So far, there have been no clinical trials using CCP in exclusively diabetic patients.

Diabetes is a pathology that has complications, including ophthalmological ones. Among the ocular alterations caused, keratoconjunctivitis sicca is very common, causing problems in the patient's daily life. As diabetics are patients with significant dry eye morbidity, where severe cases are generally refractory to conventional medication, this study aims to investigate the effectiveness of

CCP treatment in this group, given that studies in the literature have shown significant results in dry eye of other etiologies (HESS, 2015).

CHAPTER 2

OBJECTIVES

2.1 General objective:

Observe the therapeutic response of CCP in diabetic patients with symptomatic dry eye.

2.2 Specific objectives:

- To describe the epidemiological profile of patients with diabetes and dry eye treated with CCP;
- To check the frequency of cases of symptomatic dry eye (moderate to severe) in diabetic patients;
- To analyse the severity of dry eye in diabetic patients before and after the use of CCP.

CHAPTER 3

HYPOTHESIS

The use of CCP in symptomatic dry eye in diabetics who are refractory to conventional therapy is effective both in terms of symptoms (between 70 and 100 per cent) and clinical signs, and reduces the complications inherent in this disease.

CHAPTER 4

LITERATURE REVIEW

4.1 Diabetes Mellitus and its ocular manifestations

Diabetes is a group of metabolic diseases that are manifested by hyperglycaemia and generally lead to dysfunction and insufficiency of various organs, especially vascular alterations in the eyes, kidneys, nerves, brain and heart. It occurs due to defects in the secretion and/or action of insulin, the pathogenesis of which involves destruction of the beta cells of the pancreas (which produce insulin), resistance to the action of insulin, disorders of insulin secretion, among others (PORTAL BRASIL, 2014).

The number of patients with diabetes in the world was estimated at 250 million in 2012 (PORTAL BRASIL, 2014), and is expected to reach 350 million by 2025 (MINISTÉRIO DA SÁUDE, 2006). Its incidence has been increasing in developing countries and it is estimated that there will be a 60 per cent increase in prevalence in the adult population over the age of 30 by 2025, with it being more common in the 45 to 64 age group, around 11 per cent over the age of 40 in the Brazilian population (MARASCHIN et al., 2010).

According to the Ministry of Health, there are more than 10 million diabetics in Brazil, and of these, approximately 33 per cent are between the ages of 60 and 79 (MINISTÉRIO DA SÁUDE, 2006).

The diagnosis of DM2 can be established on the basis of one of the following criteria: -fasting glycaemia (8 hours) 126 mg/dl (2 measurements); glycaemia of 200 mg/dl 120 minutes after oral overload of 75 g of anhydrous glucose; or glycaemia of 200 mg/dl in a casual measurement (without considering the last meal) in an individual with symptoms suggestive of the diagnosis (polyuria, polydipsia, weight loss) (AMERICAN DIABETES ASSOCIATION, 2015).

Ocular pathologies caused by diabetes are the main cause of blindness in developed countries. These include myopia or other refractive errors, neuropathies and keratopathies, cataracts, glaucoma, vascular occlusions, diabetic retinopathy and others (JEGANATHAN; WANG; WONG, 2008; NEGI; VERNON, 2003).

The cornea, one of the most affected segments, suffers altered sensitivity due to neuropathy and can develop into keratitis, neurotrophic ulcers, secondary infections, even eye perforations and corneal scars that lead to loss of visual acuity (NEGI; VERNON, 2003).

The lens can also be affected due to acute metabolic decompensation, when there is an accumulation of sorbitol that leads to its swelling, consequently altering its dioptric power and causing hyperopia. Diabetics can also develop cataracts earlier. Type I diabetics develop a typical cortical snowflake cataract. Type II diabetics can have any type, but the subcapsular type is very common (NEGI; VERNON, 2003).

There are also peculiarities to phacectomy, which is cataract extraction surgery. These patients have more risks, such as infection, macular oedema, more inflammation, delayed healing and a worsening of diabetic retinopathy (NEGI; VERNON, 2003; JEGANATHAN; WANG; WONG, 2008).

Diabetic patients are even more at risk of developing open-angle glaucoma, closed-angle glaucoma due to the enlargement of the lens or an acute hyperglycaemic crisis causing lenticular oedema; and neovascular glaucoma, as neovascularisation occurs in the angle and iris due to the stimulation of the ischaemic retina (NEGI; VERNON, 2003; JEGANATHAN; WANG; WONG, 2008).

Among the neuro-ophthalmological manifestations, diabetes can lead to pupillary abnormalities due to autonomic neuropathy that leads to denervation of the pupil dilator and sphincter muscles, contributing to pupils that do not respond well to mydriatic drugs (NEGI; VERNON, 2003).

DM causes oculo-motor paresis in 25-30% of people over the age of 45. These are usually isolated paresis of the III, IV or VI pairs and arise due to microvascular occlusion. One of the symptoms is binocular diplopia. Spontaneous recovery is usually observed within three months, although recurrence can occur (NEGI; VERNON, 2003; JEGANATHAN; WANG; WONG, 2008).

It is also estimated that 25% of diabetic individuals may also suffer from anterior ischaemic optic neuropathy, the signs and symptoms of which are sudden visual impairment with relative afferent pupillary defect and oedema of the optic disc (NEGI; VERNON, 2003; JEGANATHAN; WANG; WONG, 2008).

It is estimated that the number of people at risk of developing sight loss as a result of diabetes will double in the next 30 years (SERRARBASSA; DIAS; VIEIRA, 2008). The World Health Organisation (WHO) estimated in 1997 that after 15 years of the disease, 2% of affected individuals will be blind and 10% will have severe visual impairment (NEGI; VERNON, 2003; JEGANATHAN; WANG; WONG, 2008).

Diabetic retinopathy (DR) is a very common complication of diabetes and is present to some degree in people who have had the disease for more than 15 years. It is considered the main cause of legal blindness in adults of working age (SERRARBASSA; DIAS; VIEIRA, 2008; BOSCO et al., 2005).

One of the earliest clinical signs in DR is increased vascular permeability, with changes in vascular endothelial growth factor (VEGF), due to the breakdown of the blood-retinal barrier, which causes macular oedema, the main cause of poor visual acuity in diabetics (BOSCO et al., 2005; SHRESTHA, 2011).

Retinopathy can be non-proliferative or proliferative. Non-proliferative retinopathy is characterised by the presence and extent of intraretinal haemorrhages, microaneurysms, venous coiling and intraretinal microvascular abnormalities (IRMA). In mild to moderate non-proliferative retinopathy, there are few small intraretinal haemorrhages and microaneurysms, minimal venous alterations and IRMA. In severe non-proliferative retinopathy, there is increased ischaemia (SERRARBASSA; DIAS; VIEIRA, 2008; BOSCO et al., 2005).

Proliferative retinopathy is characterised by neovascularisation and the absence or presence of vitreous or pre-retinal haemorrhage, the latter being more severe, and can evolve with fibrovascular proliferation and retinal detachment, resulting in visual loss (SHRESTHA, 2011). One of the main treatments for proliferative retinopathy is argon laser panphotocoagulation and the use of anti-VEGF (vascular endothelial growth factor) injections, or corticosteroids such as triamcinolone in cases of retinal oedema (FERRIS, 1996).

Dry eye is another very common complication of diabetes. It is estimated that between 8 and 54 per cent of diabetic patients have dry eye. These patients, when not diagnosed and treated appropriately, develop neurotrophic corneal ulcers, infections, leucomas, ocular perforation, and can reach blindness (MOSS; KLEIN; KLEIN, 2004; MOSS; KLEIN; KLEIN, 2008; MOSS; KLEIN; KLEIN, 2000; MANAVIAT et al., 2008).

4.2 Dry eyes

Tears have several important functions, such as lubricating the eye, transporting oxygen and carbon dioxide and other metabolites, protecting against infections and toxicity, eliminating waste that is harmful to the eye and keeping the corneal surface regular and stable, among others. It is rich in lysozymes, immunoglobulins, growth factors and vitamin A (YANG et al., 1997).

The tear film is divided into three layers. The lipid layer, secreted by the Zeiss, Meibomius and Moll glands located in the eyelids, protects the tear from evaporation and keeps it less tense to better lubricate the ocular surface (YANG et al., 1997).

The mucin layer is manufactured by the glands of Manz, crypts of Henle, epithelial cells corneal and conjunctival goblet cells and lies between the hydrophobic ocular surface and the aqueous hydrophilic film of the tear (XU et al., 1995).

The aqueous layer accounts for more than 99 per cent of the tear film; it is the thickest and most important layer, produced by the main and accessory lacrimal glands (Krause and Wolfring) (FRIDMAN, 2004).

Therefore, when there is an imbalance in any of these functional layers of the tear, dry eye syndrome can occur (YANG et al., 1997; XU et al., 1995).

According to recent consensus, dry eye or keratoconjunctivitis sicca is a multifactorial disease of the tears and ocular surface that results in discomfort, visual disturbances and instability of the tear film, with potential damage to the ocular surface (DRY EYE WORKSHOP, 2007a). It is accompanied by increased osmolarity of the tear film and inflammation of the ocular surface (TOMLINSON et al., 2006; MURUBE, 2006).

It is a common disorder, affecting a significant percentage of the population, mainly adults over 40 and women. Although some studies show no disparity in prevalence between the sexes (GUO et al., 2010; TIAN et al., 2009), a large number of them show a predominance of dry eye in women (GALOR et al., 2011; GAYTON, 2009).

The prevalence is similar all over the world, with rates varying between 7% and 33% (SCHEIN et al., 1999; MUNOZ B et al., 2000). The discrepancy observed in the literature is probably due to the absence of a consensus on the diagnosis of dry eye and the lack of standardisation of the methodology applied in research and the parameters used to classify the disease (BREWITT; SISTANI, 2001).

The difficulties in assessing dry eye begin with the divergences between the various definitions found in the literature. At the time of Hippocrates, the term xerophthalmia (from the Greek: dry eye) meant severe dry eye associated with blindness. In the last century, dry eye was restricted to Sjogren's syndrome, while other pathologies and etiologies remained unknown. Fifty years ago, von Roth introduced the term dry eye in relation to any quantitative tear deficiency; today, dry eye is understood as quantitative or compositional tear deficiencies (MURUBE et al., 2003). Scarpi suggests that the syndrome is associated with abnormalities in the relationship between tear production and the maintenance of the corneal-conjunctival surface (BELFORT JR; KARA-JOSE, 1997).

Lemp argues that dry eye is associated with a deficiency in tear production and/or an excess in tear evaporation, causing ocular discomfort and damage especially to the surface interpalpebral or beyond. He also adds that the absence of symptoms does not exclude the diagnosis of dry eye as long as there are clinical signs of lacrimal instability or alterations to the ocular surface, and that dry eye can occur without damage to the ocular surface, with only the typical symptoms and signs of lacrimal instability (LEMP, 1995).

Gomes et al. define the syndrome as a decrease in quantity, change in quality and/or decrease in tear stability (PEREIRA GOMES; LIMA; ADAN, 1999). Naranjo conceptualises dry eye as a syndrome with signs and symptoms directly related to the absence or poor quality of one or more components of the tear film (NARANJO, 2000).

Stern et al. emphasise that dry eye is caused by dysfunctions of the ocular surface, the main or accessory lacrimal glands, the meibomian glands or the neural connections that interconnect them (STERN et al., 1998). Murube defines the syndrome as a mismatch between the quality or composition of the tear and the needs of the ocular surface. The author even suggests replacing the term "dry eye" with "tear dysfunction" (MURUBE, 2000).

The main alteration in the pathophysiology of dry eye is hyperosmolarity. It occurs either due to excess evaporation of the aqueous layer or a decrease in tear secretion. It is referred to as an important parameter for the diagnosis of dry eye and is recognised as a pro-inflammatory stimulus in the development of the disease. It involves the MAP kinase and NFkB pathway and the production of inflammatory cytokines, as well as metalloproteinases (DE PAIVA et al., 2006). It results in abnormal differentiation and accelerated loss of ocular surface epithelial cells, including goblet cells, leading to film instability due to the absence of the glycocalyx produced by these cells, with consequent loss of the hydrophilic layer on the corneal surface and alteration in the antimicrobial barrier. In addition, the loss of epithelial cells leaves the corneal nerve endings exposed to environmental insults, leading to chronic ocular discomfort (FARRIS, 1994).

Inflammation of the ocular surface can be both a cause and a consequence of dry eye: dysfunction of the lacrimal glands alters the composition of the tear, leading to a state of hyperosmolarity and stimulating the production of inflammatory mediators, which in turn lead to dysfunction of the secretory glands. The inflammatory process can also be triggered by chronic irritative stress, such as wearing contact lenses, and systemic autoimmune diseases (FONSECA; ARRUDA; ROCHA, 2010). In the early stages of dry eye, alteration of the ocular surface caused by osmotic, mechanical or inflammatory stress leads to reflex stimulation of the lacrimal gland via the trigeminal nerve, causing an increase in tear secretion and blink rate to compensate. If the lacrimal gland is insufficient, as in Sjogren's Syndrome and not Sjogren's, then this will not occur, aggravating the dry eye. In evaporative dry eye, the surface disease probably leads to reduced corneal sensitivity, which fails to activate the tear reflex stimulus and the disease worsens (DRY EYE WORKSHOP, 2007a).

Another currently recognised factor in the pathogenesis of dry eye is oxidative stress, with the release of free radicals and reactive oxygen species that can cause apoptosis and cell necrosis. Oxidative stress has been associated with various systemic conditions, such as neurodegenerative diseases, cardiovascular diseases and cancer, as well as acting in eye diseases such as age-related macular degeneration, cataracts, uveitis, retinopathy of prematurity and corneal alterations (WAKAMATSU; DOGRU; TSUBOTA, 2008).

There are several risk factors for dry eye, which are also highly controversial. The DEWS separates these factors as the most relevant, where most epidemiological studies show a correlation, such as: female gender, post-menopausal oestrogen therapy, diet low in amino acids such as omega 6, post-operative refractive surgery, vitamin A deficiency, use of some medications such as antihistamines, hepatitis C, and radiotherapy; other factors are categorised as suggestive, such as Asian race, use of antidepressants, beta-blockers, diuretics, diabetes, HIV and HTLV1 infection, chemotherapy, use of isotretinoic acid, large extracapsular facectomy incisions, environments with low humidity, ovarian dysfunction and sarcoidosis; finally, there are the risk factors considered "uncertain", such as Hispanic ethnicity, smoking, alcohol, use of anxiolytics and antipsychotics, menopause, use of botulinum toxin, contraceptives, acne, pregnancy and gout (DRY EYE WORKSHOP, 2007b). An example of this controversy is evidenced in a cohort study carried out by Moss et al, with 3722 participants, which showed that a history of arthritis, smoking, caffeine use, thyroid disease, a history of gout and high cholesterol had a significant association with dry eye, while body mass, blood pressure, white blood cell count, osteoporosis, stroke, haematocrit, cardiovascular disease, allergy, use of antihistamines, parasympathomimetics, antidepressants, diuretics, antiemetics, or any other drug that had a dry eye effect, were not statistically significant in the correlation with dry eye. Alcohol consumption, the presence of eye diseases such as cataracts, macular degeneration and facectomy surgery were also not significant (MOSS; KLEIN; KLEIN, 2000).

4.2.1 The classification of dry eye

Two widely used forms of classification are the Madrid classification and the Delphi report panel.

The Madrid triple classification was created in 2003, at the 14th Congress of the European

Ophthalmological Society, through a multicentre study, based on three parameters: etiology, histopathology and clinical severity of dry eye (MURUBE et al., 2003).

The aetiological classification classifies the disease into dacryo-exocrine causes (neurological, traumatic, digenetic, inflammatory and tantalising) and pan-exocrine causes (age-related dry eye, hormonal, pharmacological, hyponutritional, immunological).

The histopathological classification is subdivided into aqueous deficiency, lipid deficiency, mucous deficiency, epitheliopathy and non-ocular causes. Hence the acronym "ALMEN" (MURUBE et al., 2003).

The classification of the clinical severity of dry eye, which ranges from grade 1 (where the patient is generally asymptomatic) to grade 3 "plus" (where the patient has constant symptoms and severe corneal damage with reduced visual acuity) (MURUBE et al., 2003).

The Delphi panel was a consensus created with the participation of a group of dry eye specialists. The classification proposed and for some time used was based on the absence or presence of eyelid disease, and the definition presented was to change dry eye disease to dysfunctional tear syndrome. This group also created a severity classification based on the patient's signs and symptoms (BEHRENS et al., 2006).

In 2007, the Dry Eye Workshop (DEWS) committee met and modified the definition of "dry eye disease", synonymous with keratoconjunctivitis sicca. It suggested not using the classification based on the absence or presence of eyelid pathology. It maintained the previous classification from 1995, which subdivides dry eye into two broad categories: dry eye due to aqueous tear deficiency and evaporative dry eye; and adapted the severity classification from the Delphi panel (LEMP, 1995).

The DEWS classification divides dry eye into the above categories: dry eye due to aqueous tear deficiency and evaporative dry eye (DRY EYE WORKSHOP, 2007a). (Figure 1)

Firstly, we list the factors that can influence a patient's risk of dry eye. These factors can be "internal" or "external". Internal factors are, for example, constitutional factors such as a wider palpebral fissure that can increase the risk of dry eye, a decreased blink rate for physiological, psychological or occupational reasons, hormone levels such as a decrease in androgens and an increase in estrogen, and the use of medication are also considered internal factors (DRY EYE WORKSHOP, 2007a).

External factors are environmental or occupational, such as places with low humidity, working in an air-conditioned environment, or people exposed to a lot of air travel, or those who work with computers, where the blink rate decreases, among others (DRY EYE WORKSHOP, 2007a).

With regard to the two broad categories of dry eye, aqueous deficiency dry eye occurs due to a decrease in secretion, both by the lacrimal gland and by conjunctival cells. Evaporative dry eye is further subdivided into those caused by the influence of external or environmental factors, and those caused by internal factors such as eyelid and ocular surface alterations (DRY EYE WORKSHOP, 2007a).

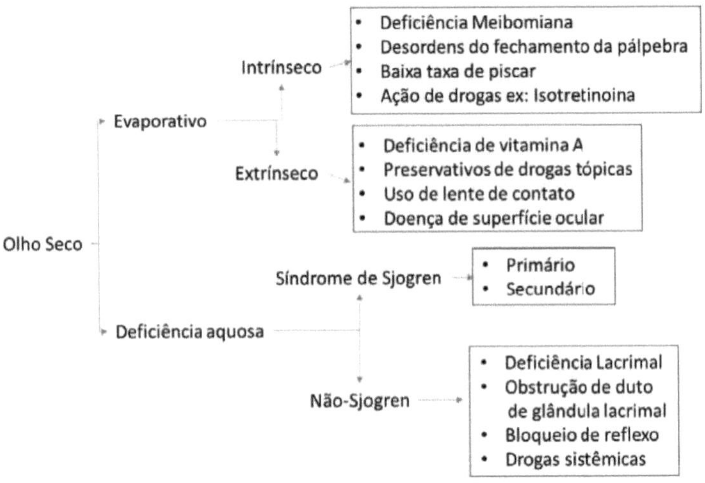

Figure 1. Classification of dry eye
Legend: classification according to the two main categories of dry eye Source: The definition and classification of dry eye disease, DEWS; 2007.

Dry eye in general can still have several associated causes, which makes diagnosis and treatment more difficult, worsening the severity of some cases.

I) Dry eye due to aqueous tear deficiency

Reduced tear secretion causes hyperosmolarity, which stimulates a cascade of inflammatory events involving MAP kinases and the NFkB pathway, generating inflammatory cytokines such as interleukin 1, TNF (tumour necrosis factor) and MMP-9 (extracellular matrix metalloproteinase). When there is inflammation or infiltration of the lacrimal gland, the inflammatory mediators come out in the tear onto the ocular surface. But there is no way of determining whether these mediators originated in the lacrimal gland or on the ocular surface itself (DE PAIVA et al., 2006).

There is controversy as to whether or not there is greater evaporation in cases of dry eye due to lacrimal deficiency, as some evidence shows that there is a decrease in the lipid layer in these patients, which could increase the evaporation rate (DRY EYE WORKSHOP, 2007a).

Dry eye due to lacrimal deficiency is subdivided into Sjogren's dry eye and non-Sjogren's dry eye.

Sjogren's syndrome (SS) is an exocrinopathy in which there is a deficiency of tear secretion due to an autoimmune process that affects the lacrimal and salivary glands and other organs in the body. The glands are infiltrated by activated T cells, which causes cell death in the acini and ducts, leading to hyposecretion (DRY EYE WORKSHOP, 2007a).

Secondary SS presents characteristics of primary SS together with the characteristics of an autoimmune type of collagen disease, such as rheumatoid arthritis, which is the most common, or systemic lupus erythematosus, polyarteritis nodosa, Wegener's granulomatosis, systemic sclerosis, biliary sclerosis, among others (DRY EYE WORKSHOP, 2007a).

Non-Sjogren's syndrome includes all causes in which lacrimal dysfunction occurs without the interference of any autoimmune factor. These are primary causes of lacrimal gland dysfunction (age-related dry eye, congenital alacrimia, familial dysautonomia), secondary causes of lacrimal gland dysfunction (sarcoidosis, lymphoma, AIDS, ablation or denervation of the gland), obstruction of the lacrimal ducts (pemphigus, trachoma, erythema multiforme, chemical burns), reflex hyposecretion (trigeminal lesion, diabetes, neurotrophic keratopathy, use of contact lenses), blockage of the motor reflex due to lesion of the VII pair, use of medication (beta-blockers, antihistamines, antispasmodics, diuretics; tricyclic antidepressants, some psychotropic drugs. Angiotensin-converting enzyme inhibitors have been shown to be a protective factor for dry eye, and calcium channel blockers and oral lipid-lowering agents have not been shown to be related to tear secretion (MOSS; KLEIN; KLEIN, 2004; SCHEIN et al., 1999)). Evaporative dry eye occurs due to excessive evaporative loss of the aqueous layer. The causes can be intrinsic or extrinsic. Intrinsic causes include meibomian gland dysfunctions, eyelid opening disorders, ocular exposure such as exophthalmos and lagophthalmos, decreased blinking rate, among others. Extrinsic causes include ocular surface disorders such as hypovitaminosis A which leads to xerophthalmia, chronic use of anaesthetic eye drops or others with preservatives such as antiglaucoma eye drops (TEI et al., 2000; PISELLA; POULIQUEN; BAUDOUIN, 2002; PHARMAKAKIS et al., 2002), the use of contact lenses and allergic conjunctivitis, which also greatly alters the ocular surface (FUJISHIMA et al., 1996).

4.2.2 Classification based on the severity of dry eye

This was adapted and modified by the DEWS *(Dry Eye Workshop)* from the scheme proposed by the Delphi panel (DRY EYE WORKSHOP, 2007a; BEHRENS et al., 2006). It consists of classifying dry eye into grades 1 to 4 (mild to severe), which is based on the frequency or intensity with which the following criteria occur: ocular discomfort (dry eye symptoms), visual disturbances, corneal and conjunctival colouration, conjunctival injection, tear alterations, meibomian dysfunction, *But time (Break up time)* or tear film *break up* time (TRFL), and Schirmer's test (Table 1).

Table 1. DEWS severity classification

Categorisation of dry eye severity (based on DEWS)

Severity of dry eye	1	2	3	4
Discomfort, severity and frequency	Mild and/or episodic; occurs under environmental stress	Moderate or chronic episodic; with or without stress	Severe frequent or constant; no stress	Severe and/or disabling and constant
Visual symptoms	Absent or mild episodic	Annoying or limiting activities; episodic	Annoying, limiting activities constantly and/or chronically	Constant and/or possibly disabling
Conjunctival injection	Absent or mild	Absent or mild	+/-	+/++
Conjunctival colouring	Absent or mild	Variable	Moderate to severe	Accentuated
Corneal colouring	Absent or mild	Variable	Accentuated centre	Severe punctate erosions
Corneal and tear signs	Absent or mild	Mild debris, meniscus reduction	Filamentary wax, adhesion of mucus, increase in tear debris	Filamentary keratitis, mucus adhesion, increased tear ducts, ulceration
Eyelids/Meibomian glands	DGM* variably present	DGM* variably present	Frequent	Trichiasis, keratinisation, symblepharon
TFBUT**	Variable	<10	<5	Immediate
Schirmer (mm/5min)	Variable	<10	<5	<2

*LGD = lacrimal gland dysfunction

**TFBUT=tear film break-up ti me (tear film break-up time)

Caption: Classification of dry eye severity, graded from 1 to 4

Source: Fonseca, E.C., Arruda, G. V., Rocha, E. M. Dry eye: etiopathogenesis and treatment Arq. Bras. Oftalmol. 2010;73(2):197-203.

4.2.3 Clinical and laboratory diagnosis of dry eye

There is no diagnostic standardisation for dry eye, and the literature emphasises the lack of correlation between one objective test and another, and also between the tests and the patient's symptoms. This is probably due to the heterogeneous causes of dry eye and the difficulty in understanding the pathophysiology of this disease (ALVES et al., 2014).

A recent 2007 evaluation by the American Academy of Ophthalmology established guidelines for dealing with dry eye (AMERICAN ACADEMY OF OPHTHALMOLOGY, 2013), which consist of a good clinical history, a general clinical examination to detect whether there are systemic diseases (such as rheumatic diseases) or other conditions, an external ocular examination of the eyelids, skin, nerves, visual acuity and biomicroscopy.

The history mainly includes the patient's complaints related to dry eye, which are: heaviness in the eyelids, burning, itching, eye irritation, foreign body sensation, photophobia, dryness, blurred vision, tearing, among others. These worsen during the day, with exposure to cold air or smoke, pollution, prolonged computer use, wearing contact lenses and staying in a dry environment. Characterising the symptoms and the effect of topical medications in these cases is necessary. The most common symptom in dry eye has been ocular "fatigue", reported in more than 70 per cent of cases (AMERICAN ACADEMY OF OPHTHALMOLOGY, 2013).

Therefore, in the ocular history, it is important to remember to investigate allergic conjunctivitis, contact lens use, previous ocular surgeries such as cataracts, refractive surgeries, corneal transplants, blepharoplasties and other eyelid surgeries, diseases that affect the ocular surface such as herpes, ocular pemphigus, Stevens-Jonhsons (AMERICAN ACADEMY OF OPHTHALMOLOGY, 2013).

In the systemic assessment, it is necessary to check if the patient is a smoker or is exposed to any type of pollutant at work, if they have any dermatological diseases such as rosacea. Check eyelash and eyelid hygiene, presence of atopic disease, menopause, systemic inflammatory disease such as lupus, arthritis, scleroderma, lymphoma, sarcoidosis, among others.

It's a good idea to take note of the medications you use, as several classes can cause dry eye in some cases (antihistamines, diuretics, hormones and hormone antagonists, antidepressants, antiarrhythmic medications, isotretinoin, diphenoxylate/atropine, beta-adrenergic antagonists, chemotherapy agents and any other drug with an anticholinergic effect) (AMERICAN ACADEMY OF OPHTHALMOLOGY, 2013).

It is also pertinent to assess previous history of trauma, such as chemical trauma, chronic viral infections (e.g. hepatitis C, human immunodeficiency virus), non-ocular surgery (e.g. bone marrow transplant, head and neck surgery, surgery for trigeminal neuralgia), radiotherapy (of the orbit), neurological conditions (Parkinson's disease, Bell's palsy, trigeminal neuralgia), oral diseases with dry mouth or oral ulcers, among other systemic diseases (AMERICAN ACADEMY OF OPHTHALMOLOGY, 2013).

Validated questionnaires such as the OSDI (Ocular Surface Disease Index-Allergan) (SCHIFFMAN et al., 2000), the DEQ (Dry Eye Questionaire) (BEGLEY et al., 2002) and the McMonnies Questionaire (NICHOLS; NICHOLS; MITCHELL, 2004), among others, are recommended for assessing dry eye. These often don't correlate with objective tests and should be used in conjunction with other clinical history data.

After carrying out an ophthalmological examination, with visual acuity, biomicroscopy (of the eyelids, tear ducts, eyelashes, conjunctiva and cornea), external examination (assessing proptosis, exophthalmos, how the skin, hands, and the function of the cranial nerve pairs are) and fundoscopy, some objective tests are used to complement the investigation, such as, the patient's blink rate, which is generally reduced, visual acuity, assessment of the height of the tear meniscus (less than 0.35mm is abnormal), the quality of the tear film (if there is mucus or debris), tests to check for changes in the ocular surface, tear clearance rate, corneal stoichiometry, corneal topography, among others (FRIDMAN, 2004).

Diagnostic tests for dry eye are generally not fully objective, they don't correlate with the patient's symptoms, nor is there a consensus on which would be the best diagnostic combination. However, the DEWS suggests a combination that is widely used in clinical practice, with good sensitivity and accuracy, which includes the Schirmer test, corneal staining and TRFL (tear film break up time) (DRY EYE WORKSHOP, 2007c).

Tear stability: this is assessed using the (TFBUT) or tear film break-up time (TRFL), which consists of calculating how long it takes for the applied fluorescein film to break up. When the first dry spot appears after instillation, the time is noted. Several authors consider values below 10 seconds to be abnormal. Authors have found a specificity of approximately 72 per cent in normal patients, and a sensitivity of 36 per cent on average in cases of mild dry eye, and approximately 60 per cent in severe dry eye. BUT can generate false results when performed inappropriately, such as in cases of too much eye drop instillation, poor eyelid closure, previous use of eye ointments, blepharitis with too much mucus on the ocular surface, alterations to the corneal epithelium, among others, which can cause artefacts (FRIDMAN, 2004).

Fluorescein staining: can be used as an alternative to rose bengal and lissamine green. This dye fills in the epithelial spaces when there is a loss of integrity (DRY EYE WORKSHOP, 2007a).

Staining with rose bengal and lissamine green: when you can't stain with fluorescein, you can try rose bengal or lissamine green (less toxic, but more difficult to find commercially). In this case, when there are changes in the mucin layer, the mucus precipitates and forms filaments that are stained with this dye. When there are changes, the conjunctiva is well coloured. Lissamine green stains devitalised proteins (QUEIROGA; DINIZ, 2010; FRIDMAN, 2004).

Schirmer test and its variants: introduced by Schirmer in 1903, it is very important in clinical practice. It translates tear aqueous deficiency. It is carried out using a standard millimetre filter paper on the lower eyelid fornix, with the eyes open or closed. After 5 minutes, the amount of moisture on the paper is measured (VAN BIJSTERVELD, 1969).

The Schirmer 1 test, which assesses basal and reflex tear secretion, is carried out without anaesthetic eye drops in a not too bright environment. After 5 minutes, values below 10mm or above 30mm are considered abnormal. According to van Bijsterveld, Schirmer values below 5mm have a sensitivity of 85% for dry eye, and specificity of 83%. When below 10mm, the specificity varies around 77% (VAN BIJSTERVELD, 1969).

In the Schirmer 2 test, a cotton swab is inserted into the nasal cavity to increase the reflex stimulus; some authors consider it abnormal when the value is less than 15mm in 5 minutes. Other authors don't consider it an important test because the reduction in reflex secretion doesn't have as much of a clinical impact on dry eye. The basal tear secretion test uses an anaesthetic to eliminate the effect of reflex secretion, with results 40% lower than Schirmer 1 (FRIDMAN, 2004).

There are also laboratory tests, which are less available in our country, sometimes expensive and their low accuracy doesn't make them as advantageous, such as research into lacrimal lysozyme and lactoferrin, evaluation of the mucin layer, lacrimal osmolarity and impression cytology (FRIDMAN, 2004).

It is the combination of anamnesis, ophthalmological examination and the results of one or more tests that can diagnose dry eye (DRY EYE WORKSHOP, 2007c). To date, there is no gold standard test for dry eye.(PAN et al., 2013) 4.3 Diabetes and dry eye

The *Beaver Dam* study showed that 18.1 per cent of diabetic patients had dry eye compared to 14.1 per cent of non-diabetics. Another similar study showed a difference of 20.6 per cent in diabetics versus 13.8 per cent in non-diabetics. Microvascular alterations in the lacrimal glands have been suggested in addition to neuropathic dysfunctions (KAISERMAN et al., 2005; MOSS; KLEIN; KLEIN, 2000; MOSS; KLEIN; KLEIN, 2004).

There are indications that diabetes, through insulin resistance and hyperglycaemia, can cause oxidative stress and dry eye. Patients with diabetes have keratopathies such as punctate keratitis, with the possibility of trophic ulcers and persistent epithelial defects, which can develop into severe complications such as corneal scars and perforations (MANAVIAT et al., 2008).

The mechanism of dry eye is probably related to autonomic dysfunction. Aldose reductase, the first enzyme in the sorbitol pathway, may also be involved. One study has already described an increase in glycosylated haemoglobin in diabetic patients with dry eye (DRY EYE WORKSHOP, 2007a).

Another study revealed that these DM patients also have decreased tear secretion and a reduced TFBUT. With regard to pathophysiology, it is believed that insulin resistance and hyperglycaemia are involved in diabetic dry eye. Hyperglycaemia and oxidative stress release advanced glycation end products, which modify the protein matrix of various tissues and activate pro-inflammatory cytokines leading to cell damage, which occurs for example in the lacrimal glands (MANAVIAT et al., 2008).

DM then causes a reduction in the tear film and its instability, as it also reduces the lipid layer of the tear, with an increase in conjunctival squamous metaplasia and a decrease in corneal sensitivity (ALVES et al., 2008).

Insulin plays an important role in metabolic and mitogenic effects in target tissues, through the mediation of nutrients, energy reserves, gene expression and protein synthesis. Exocrine secretions such as saliva, tears and milk contain insulin which participates in the metabolism and growth of these glands. In addition, the importance of insulin in the epithelial cell proliferation of glands and the cornea has also been mentioned (ALVES et al., 2008).

The prevalence of dry eye in diabetes varies in the literature. Manaviat et al showed that in 199 diabetic patients, 108 (54.3 per cent) had dry eye, which did not vary in relation to gender or age, but correlated with the duration of diabetes (MANAVIAT et al., 2008). In another study of 3,722 participants, the prevalence varied between 8 per cent and 19 per cent, increasing with age (MOSS; KLEIN; KLEIN, 2000). Another study of 140 patients revealed a difference between the sexes, with 80 per cent of dry eye in women (SENDECKA; BARYLUK; POLZ-DACEWICZ, 2004). Some authors have reported an increased incidence of dry eye in diabetic patients using medication such as diuretics, antihistamines or with other associated comorbidities (MOSS; KLEIN; KLEIN, 2004).

Hom and De Land showed that patients with a family history of diabetes were more likely to have dry eye symptoms than those without (HOM; DE LAND, 2006). Kaiserman and co-authors observed that the use of lubricants by diabetic patients was much higher than in non-diabetics, 20.6% and 13.88% respectively (KAISERMAN et al., 2005).

A study comparing diabetic and non-diabetic children, evaluating dry eye symptoms and objective tests (TBUT and Schirmer), showed that 15.4 per cent of children with type 1 diabetes complained of dry eye symptoms, and of these, 7.7 per cent had alterations in the objective tests. In contrast, of the children in the control group, only 1.9 per cent had symptoms and of these 0.9 per cent had alterations in the tests (AKINCI; CETINKAYA; AYCAN, 2007).

There are studies that show that the TFBUT is reduced in diabetics, and that the Schirmer test is also reduced when compared to control groups (GOEBBELS, 2000; JIN et al., 2003). It has also been reported that diabetic dry eye is related to diabetic retinopathy (MANAVIAT et al., 2008). In another study, no relationship was observed between dry eye and other diabetic complications, such as neuropathy and nephropathy (NAJAFI et al., 2013).

4.4 Conventional treatment

There is currently no cure for dry eye. Any causative factors that can be treated should be addressed. In mild dry eye, the important measures are environmental guidance and modifications, discontinuation of topical or systemic medications associated with worsening when possible, lubrication with artificial tears, ointment or gel and eyelid hygiene (PAN et al., 2013).

There is a wide variety of artificial tears, which differ in the electrolytes they contain, their preservatives, viscosity and osmolarity (LEMP, 1995). One study showed that artificial tears containing 1% sodium hyaluronate without preservatives have been effective in cases of dry eye, improving osmolarity, keratopathy and BUT in these patients (JONNES, 1984).

The advent of new presentations of artificial tears, also including hypotonic solutions, or containing lipids that prevent evaporation, substances with bioadhesive properties that increase water retention, formulas that contain substances that protect against cellular stress caused by the hypertonicity of the tear, represents progress in this area of treatment (ARAGONA et al., 2013), but these tears are still far from having the properties of natural tears (KLENKLER; SHEARDOWN; JONES, 2007).

For moderate dry eye, in addition to the above treatments, the following measures are appropriate: anti-inflammatory agents (topical ciclosporin and corticosteroids, systemic supplements with omega-3 fatty acids, or with linoleic or gamma linoleic acid considering their anti-inflammatory properties, less alcohol consumption and more water consumption, tear point occluders and proper glasses.

Corticosteroids have improved symptoms in some cases as they reduce inflammation (DE PAIVA et al., 2006), but their prolonged use may be related to the appearance of cataracts and increased eye pressure (BLOMQUIST, 2011). In 2002, the FDA approved cyclosporine 0.05% for use in dry eye, with good results in some cases with increased tear production (TOKER; ASFUROGLU, 2010), although adverse effects such as eye irritation can limit treatment (WANG et al., 2008).

For severe dry eye, in addition to the above treatments, the following measures are appropriate: systemic cholinergic agonists, systemic anti-inflammatory agents, mucolytic agents, tears with autologous serum, contact lenses, correction of eyelid abnormalities, permanent occlusion of the lacrimal point and tarsorrhaphy (AMERICAN ACADEMY OF OPHTHALMOLOGY, 2013).

4.5 The use of autologous serum

The most common conventional therapy used to treat dry eye is artificial tears. Unfortunately, these eye drops are devoid of substances that are essential for lubricating the eye, such as growth factors, vitamins, immunoglobulins and others present in natural tears. Another disadvantage of artificial lubricant eye drops is the preservatives they contain, which sometimes even worsen the patient's symptoms (LIU et al., 2005).

In addition, many patients, especially those with severe dry eye, do not respond well to this usual therapy. It has also been discovered that artificial tears do not maintain intracellular ATP at acceptable levels or the integrity of the cell membrane (POON et al., 2001).

Human serum or plasma is rich in epidermal growth factor, vitamin A, beta growth factor (factor-0), fibronectin and cytokines that are found in the tear, and bactericidal factors (immunoglobulins IgG, IgA, and lysozyme) that help keep the ocular surface healthy (KOFFLER, 2006).

Tear components, also present in serum, such as epidermal growth factors and vitamin A, are important for the proliferation, differentiation and maturation of the ocular surface epithelium. Studies with cultures of human corneal fibroblasts and endothelial cells show that these cells express epithelial growth factor and have their DNA synthesis increased in the presence of these factors (WOOST et al., 1992).

Of all the factors, the most important are: epithelial growth factor (EGF) which accelerates the process of epithelial cell migration, TGF-B, (fibroblast growth factor beta) which is involved in the process of stromal and epithelial healing vitamin A which prevents squamous metaplasia of the epithelium, fibronectin which promotes cell migration, albumin which has anti-apoptotic activity, a - 2 macroglobulin which has anti-collagenase action, platelet-derived growth factor (PDGF- AB) which promotes healing, hepatocyte growth factor, substance P and insulin-like growth factor which help the epithelium migrate and adhere to the stroma (LÓPEZ-GARCÍA et al., 2007).

The Ebers Papyrus, 1534 BC, is the first reference in history to the use of a blood derivative in the eye. In 1975, autologous serum was used for dry eye for the first time by Ralph et al (RALPH; DOANE; DOHLMAN, 1975).

Fox et al. reported the benefits of autologous serum in patients with Sjogren's syndrome in the 1980s, but this was only put into practice when Tsubota et al. demonstrated its efficacy in a study of 12 patients with dry eye at the end of the decade (FOX et al., 1984) (TSUBOTA et al., 1999a). During these decades, fetal bovine serum, allogeneic serum and umbilical cord serum have been used, but as they are heterologous products, they present a greater risk of allergic reactions and transmission of infectious diseases, and their use is only possible in a few specialised centres (YOON et al., 2007; SHARMA et al., 2011).

Later, several authors reported the use of autologous serum in dry eye with good results (NOBLE et al., 2004; TANANUVAT et al., 2001; HYON; LEE; YUN, 2007).

Kojima et al. compared autologous serum and commercial eye drops in patients who used them for a fortnight, six times a day. When comparing BUT (Break up time) values, it was significantly higher in the group of patients who used autologous serum (KOJIMA et al., 2005).

More recently, in 2008, Lee and Chen evaluated the long-term efficacy and safety of applying 20% autologous serum in cases of severe dry eye in 23 patients followed up for approximately 18 months. 74% of patients on average obtained an improvement in the fluorescein staining pattern, 76% reported an excellent improvement in symptoms, and there were no significant complications in this study (LEE; CHEN, 2008).

Other indications for the use of autologous serum have been epithelial defects (TSUBOTA et al., 1999b; YOUNG et al., 2004; ALVARADO VALERO et al., 2004), recurrent corneal erosions (REIDY; PAULUS; GONA, 2000; DEL CASTILLO et al., 2002), neurotrophic keratopathy (MATSUMOTO et al., 2004), trabeculectomy ampoules (MATSUO et al., 2005), superior limbic keratoconjunctivitis (GOTO et al., 2001), graft versus host disease (MIXON et al., 2014), post refractive surgery (NODA-TSURUYA et al., 2006) (JAVALOY et al., 2013), Mooren's ulcer (MAVRAKANAS; KIEL; DOSSO, 2007) and aniridia keratopathy (LÓPEZ-GARCÍA et al., 2008).

With regard to stability, Tsubota et al. reported that the concentration of growth factors and vitamin A and fibronectin in autologous serum diluted with sodium chloride and preserved at a temperature of 4 degrees lasts 1 month, and at -20 degrees lasts 3 months (TSUBOTA et al., 1999a).

Autologous serum has been well tolerated, with few complications. In the literature, rare cases of infection have been reported (LEITE et al., 2006), as well as the deposition of immunoglobulins in the cornea and keratic infiltrates in one case (MCDONNELL; SCHANZLIN; RAO, 1988). The downside is that some patients, especially those with comorbidities such as anaemia, cannot use it frequently (LÓPEZ-GARCÍA et al., 2007). In this case, there is still the option of using serum rich in growth factors obtained from the umbilical cord (VERSURA et al., 2015).

There is still no standardisation in the production of autologous serum, but it is important to stress the importance of carrying out previous serologies on patients (for hepatitis, Chagas, syphilis and Hiv) and also to use sterile conditions when preparing eye drops, and before using them the patient should submit a sample to culture for bacteria and other microorganisms (QUINTO; CAMPOS; BEHRENS, 2008).

A systematic review carried out to assess the effectiveness of autologous serum compared to commercial tears (PAN et al., 2013) evaluated four clinical trials comparing both treatments (KOJIMA et al., 2005; NODA-TSURUYA et al., 2006; TANANUVAT et al., 2001; URZUA et al., 2012). and concluded that, due to the great heterogeneity of the individuals selected, also considering the making and maintenance of the eye drops, how to use them, as well as the objective and subjective assessment of dry eye, new randomised studies are needed to standardise these items. However, based on current evidence, they observed that symptoms improved in patients who used autologous serum, but there was no significant difference in terms of improvement in objective signs.

4.6 The composition of the platelet concentrate

PC (platelet concentrate) consists of a suspension of platelets in plasma, prepared by double centrifugation of a unit of whole blood. Platelets secrete some very important growth factors for the tear, such as platelet-derived angiogenesis factor, platelet-derived epithelial growth factor and platelet factor 4 (RAZOUK; REICHE, 2004).

Epidermal (epithelial) growth factor accelerates the healing process and epithelial migration in the cornea, as well as stimulating DNA synthesis in epithelial cells and being chemotactic for human epithelial and stromal cells. This factor has an anti-apoptotic effect and has been associated with the production of mucin-1 by some conjunctival cells (LÓPEZ-PLANDOLIT et al., 2011).

Transforming growth factor b1 (TGF -b1) has its levels increased in the epithelium during stromal repair processes in the cornea. It is secreted by platelets, endothelial cells, lymphocytes and macrophages (LÓPEZ-PLANDOLIT et al., 2011).

In the cornea, TGF-b1 decreases the migration of keratocytes and favours the migration of fibroblasts and the production of extracellular matrix by a double mechanism: stimulating the production of collagen, fibronectin and proteoglycans, and decreasing their degradation by inhibiting proteolytic enzymes. Together with platelet-derived growth factor (PDGF) and integrins, it also promotes the differentiation of myofibroblasts, thus exerting an important anti-inflammatory action (LÓPEZ- GARCÍA et al., 2008).

Vitamin A is one of the main epitheliotrophic factors in autologous serum, its concentration being 100 times higher than in natural tears. It prevents squamous metaplasia of the epithelium (GEERLING; MACLENNAN; HARTWIG, 2004).

Platelet-derived growth factor was one of the first to be characterised. It is chemotactic for monocytes, macrophages and fibroblasts and stimulates the expression of other factors such as TGF-b (GEERLING; MACLENNAN; HARTWIG, 2004).

Fibronectin is a soluble protein that promotes healing and phagocytosis. On the ocular surface it is one of the main factors in corneal re-epithelialisation. It has been used, for example, in corneal ulcers and epithelial defects with good results (PHAN et al., 1991).

Annexin A5 has been investigated as an alternative to fibronectin eye drops. It interacts with the dominant kinase of some integrins, mimicking their effect. It also stimulates the secretion of plasminogen activator-type urokinase, whose expression is increased in epithelial defects, thus facilitating cell migration.

Albumin is one of the most important proteins in the blood. It reduces the natural degradation of cytokines and growth factors in areas of tissue injury and shows anti-apoptotic activity. The healing effect of this protein has already been demonstrated in vitro and in vivo (TSUBOTA et al., 1999b; UNTERLAUFT et al., 2009; SHIMMURA et al., 2003).

Alpha 2 macroglobulin neutralises proteolytic enzymes. It is useful in eye burns and marginal ulcers (TSUBOTA et al., 1999b; POON et al., 2001).

Beta fibroblast growth factor is a factor that promotes corneal healing, not only by increasing cell proliferation but also motility (ANDRESEN; EHLERS, 1998).

Insulin-like growth factor 1 helps promote epithelial cell migration (YAMADA et al., 2004). Its use has been effective in patients with neurotrophic keratopathy (YAMADA et al., 2004). Patients with seasonal and vernal conjunctivitis have shown an elevation of P-selectin in the tear. This suggests that P-selectin may be related to the pathogenesis of allergic conjunctivitis (MATSUURA et al., 2004).

Neural growth factor (NGF) is the best known neurotrophin. Some reports show its efficacy in trophic ulcers. It can also restore the function of damaged neurons. It also induces the production of SP and calcitonin generelated peptide in the central and peripheral nervous system. The effects of NGF on the ocular surface are mediated by specific receptors located on the corneal and conjunctival epithelial cells (MATSUURA et al., 2004).

4.6.1 The use of platelet concentrate in dry eye

Platelet concentrate has already been used in other medical areas such as orthopaedics, maxillofacial surgery and dermatology, among others. Platelet concentrate eye drops (POC) have higher levels of EGF (epithelial growth factor) and vitamin A than autologous serum (ANITUA et al., 2004; ANITUA et al., 2005).

Autologous serum also contains pro-inflammatory cytokines derived from leukocytes and monocytes, which can be deleterious in patients with immunological alterations or diseases (GEERLING; MACLENNAN; HARTWIG, 2004; LÓPEZ- GARCÍA et al., 2007); hence the advantage of platelet concentrate, which will not contain these inflammatory immunoglobulins. Freire et al. observed in a study that the concentrate rich in growth factors regulates the expression of various genes in cell communication and differentiation, improving the biological activity of corneal epithelial cells when compared to autologous serum (FREIRE et al., 2012).

In another study, it was observed that plasma eye drops rich in growth factors protect the ocular surface more from the formation of corneal scars and opacities due to the reduction of myofibroblasts through the induction of TGF-b1 (ANITUA; TROYA; ORIVE, 2012). Anitua et al. (2013) observed this mainly in patients who underwent PRK and reduced the incidence of haze in those who used platelet eye drops (ANITUA et al., 2013). Studies have also observed in rabbits with corneal ulcers that there was an acceleration in corneal regeneration and an improvement in collagen fibre formation in the corneal stroma (KHAKSAR et al., 2011).

It is then excellent in the corneal epithelial healing process, as it adheres to the damaged tissue, attracting cytokines and growth factors and transforming the fibroblast into fibrin, completing the repair process (ALIO et al., 2007b). It also causes a reduction in inflammation by indirect action, by reducing osmolarity, thus diluting the pro-inflammatory factors on the ocular surface. This is also due to the presence of the interleukin-1 receptor antagonist in plasma rich in growth factors, as well as the presence of metalloproteinase inhibitors (ALIO et al., 2007b).

There are also other growth factors, such as epidermal growth factor, which helps with corneal re-epithelialisation (ANITUA et al., 2004). Its use has been reported in corneal ulcers (KIM; SHIN; KIM, 2012; REZENDE et al., 2007; ALIO; RODRIGUEZ; WRÓBELDUDZINSKA, 2015), in chemical burns (PANDA et al., 2012; MARQUEZ DE ARACENA DEL CID; MONTERO DE ESPINOSA ESCORIAZA, 2009), in ocular surface syndrome after refractive surgery (JAVALOY et al., 2013), in a case of lacrimal function restoration, 2013), in a case of lacrimal function restoration (MY, 2014), in blepharoplasty surgeries (VICK et al., 2006), in cases of ocular surface diseases such as graft versus host (PEZZOTTA et al., 2012) and recently Alio et al. demonstrated in a study of 18 patients with severe dry eye that 89 per cent obtained symptom improvement with platelet concentrate eye drops (ALIO et al., 2007a).

Lopez-Plandolit et al. carried out a prospective study of 16 patients with moderate to severe dry eye, refractory to conventional medications, and observed a statistically significant improvement in the patients who used plasma rich in growth factors, but no significant change in the impression cytologies of these patients (LÓPEZ-PLANDOLIT et al., 2011).

4.6.2 Methods for obtaining platelet concentrate eye drops

The two main methods of obtaining platelets are by autologous donation and by the platelet apheresis technique. The advantage of the apheresis technique is that the concentration of platelets is higher in the final concentrate, which must contain at least 5.5×10^{10} platelets, while its disadvantage is the cost, which is extremely higher than the total autologous donation technique (RAZOUK; REICHE, 2004).

In the apheresis technique for collecting platelets, Rezende et al. used the Haemonetics MCS+ 9000 automatic cell separator and the specific 995-E apheresis platelet kit (Haemonetics Corp.). In this system, through a venipuncture, the patient's own blood is drained into a separation device. An optical refraction analyser separates the platelet layer and the remaining blood is completely returned to the patient, determining the end of a cycle. Sodium citrate can be used as an anticoagulant at a rate of one for every 9 ml of whole blood processed. In two cycles, 72 ml of platelet concentrate are collected, and the patient's haematimetric indices are assessed before and after the procedure, as well as the platelet concentrate (Coulter - ActDiff) (REZENDE et al., 2007).

Platelet growth factors are generally obtained in a classified room, which is why the platelet concentrate was handled in a category II-Type A biological safety cabinet. Then 2800 microlitres of 10% calcium chloride were added to the platelet concentrate, and the final product was kept at +37 degrees Celsius for approximately 30 minutes (REZENDE et al., 2007).

The unit was then centrifuged (900G) and the supernatant serum, which contains the platelet growth factors, was transferred to four 50 ml falcon tubes (Becton-Dickinson) and kept at -80 degrees Celsius (Revco). Aerobic and anaerobic bacteria and fungal agents were systematically analysed (REZENDE et al., 2007).

In the study by Rezende et al., the serum with platelet growth factors was released as follows: every week, 01 falcon tube containing approximately 10 ml of autologous serum with platelet growth factors was defrosted and transferred to cholera bottles. The patient was instructed to keep the biological medicine at a temperature below -10 degrees Celsius (freezer) and to defrost it naturally immediately before each use (REZENDE et al., 2007).

Alio et al. used the autologous donation technique to obtain platelets, when patients underwent venipuncture and 80 to 100 ml of blood was collected in sterile 10 ml tubes containing 1 ml of sodium citrate to prevent clotting. These tubes were left at room temperature for ten minutes and only the supernatant (upper fraction of the tube) was collected as the final product. The platelet concentrate was then prepared under sterile conditions in a laminar flow room. Two to three millilitres of this concentrate was then placed in sterile eye drops. The eye drop bottles were kept at -20 degrees Celsius, and only when the patient was going to use an eye drop bottle did he defrost it, then keep it at +4 degrees Celsius, discarding this bottle at the end of a week, when he defrosted a new one (ALIO et al., 2007a.).

Both methods require the patient to donate autologous blood. Autologous blood does not transmit diseases, there are no haemolytic reactions (alloimmunisation), allergic reactions, immunological reactions (immunomodulation) or acute lung damage from the transfusion, which are common complications in heterologous donations (VANE; GANEM, 2006).

Contraindications for autologous donations are anaemia or other types of pathological haemodilution, conditions that cause a drop in oxygen and haemoglobin saturation (less than 11mg/dl), liver diseases, nephropathies, coagulopathies, haemoglobinopathies, decompensated heart diseases, the presence of infectious diseases such as Chagas, syphilis, HIV, HTLV, hepatitis B and C, and other blood-borne diseases are considered "relative" contraindications, since the patient is the one who will receive it, but the healthcare team may be contaminated when handling this blood, and in the case of HIV, there may be reactivation of the virus when it is reinfused (VANE; GANEM, 2006; SÍRIO LIBANÊS HOSPITAL, 2010).

Complications of autologous donation are those inherent to a donor, such as hypotension, anaemia, angina and contamination of the blood bag material (VANE; GANEM, 2006).

CHAPTER 5

METHOD

5.1 Type of study

The study design was an open, prospective, non-randomised, time series clinical trial.

5.2 Study site

Dr Alberto Antunes University Hospital and João Paulo II Basic Health Unit, Maceió-Alagoas-Brazil.

5.3 Research Ethics Committee approval

The project was approved by the Research Ethics Committee (CEP) of the Federal University of Alagoas, and by the National Research Ethics Committee (CONEP) (Annex A). It was also registered with the Brazilian Registry of Clinical Trials (REBEC) (Annex A). The recommendations of the Declaration of Helsinki were followed (WORLD MEDICAL ASSOCIATION, 2013).

5.4 Sample

5.4.1 Inclusion criteria

Symptomatic dry eye, moderate to severe (at least one symptom and one sign from grades 2 to 4) classified using the Dry Eye Workshop severity table (DRY EYE WORKSHOP, 2007a) which is based on the Delphi Panel (BEHRENS et al., 2006) (Figure 2), refractory or with low responsiveness to conventional therapy.

5.4.2 Exclusion criteria

Patients with keratopathies, active eye infections, eye allergies, a history of refractive surgery, the use of contact lenses, the use of glaucoma eye drops, corticosteroids or antibiotics, a diagnosis of previous rheumatic disease, as well as those with contraindications to undergoing autologous donation were excluded, such as blood-borne diseases (positive serology), heart disease, nephropathy, liver disease, coagulopathy, recent stroke (less than 6 months), anaemia with haemoglobin less than 11mg/dl, haematocrit less than 33%, infections or neoplasms, and patients who did not have adequate venous access to perform the technique.

Individuals under the age of 18, the mentally disabled, pregnant women, indigenous people and foreigners were also excluded.

5.4.3 Sampling

5.4.3.1 Patient identification

We assessed 221 diabetic patients diagnosed according to the ADA criteria (AMERICAN DIABETES ASSOCIATION, 2015), from the University Hospital of Alagoas and the João Paulo II

Basic Reference Unit, in Maceió-Alagoas-Brazil, with clinical follow-up through the endocrinology and medical clinic sectors, and referred to the ophthalmology sector. They were approached by the examining ophthalmologist about whether they had any ocular complaints of dry eye, then informed about the research and asked if they were interested in undergoing a new treatment.

Patients' clinical data was collected, such as identification, co-existing diseases, use of medication and eye drops, pathologies, previous eye surgeries or treatments, personal history such as smoking, using a questionnaire (Appendix A) or data already in medical records.

5.4.3.2 Patient selection

Patients with moderate to severe dry eye who were refractory or unresponsive to conventional therapy were selected.

5.5 Informed consent form

Only the patients selected for CCP treatment who accepted and showed interest in taking part in the study signed the Informed Consent Form (ICF), which was given to them at the time of the primary ophthalmological consultation (prior to treatment) (Appendix B).

5.6 Variables

5.6.1 Primary variables: Symptomatology and clinical signs of dry eye.

5.6.2 Secondary variables: Symptoms of ocular discomfort (dryness, stinging, burning, blurred vision, eyes sticking together or with mucus or crusts), conjunctival injection, conjunctival and corneal colouring, meibomian dysfunction, eyelid changes, tear and ocular surface changes, Schirmer's test, tear film break-up time (TRFL) or BUT (Break Up Time) test and visual acuity.

5.6.3 Additional data: age, gender, ethnicity, duration of diabetes, average fasting glycaemia.

5.6.4 Measurement of variables

It was carried out using the DEWS (DRY EYE WORKSHOP, 2007a) dry eye severity classification table (figure 2), which follows the Delphi Panel, in which one sign and one symptom from each level is enough to correspond to it (BEHRENS et al., 2006).

1.Symptoms:

a) Evaluation of ocular discomfort (symptoms such as stinging, burning, foreign body sensation, dryness, itching, mucousy eyes, among others), using a specific questionnaire (Appendix A) graded from 1 to 4, where "1" means that the discomfort occurs rarely or not at all, and the frequency increases up to level "4" where the complaint occurs almost constantly. We identified the typical symptoms of dry eye in isolation, characterising "ocular discomfort", but in the final score we chose the symptom with the highest gradation;

b) Visual clouding, also graded from 1 to 4, also according to the intensity of this symptom and its frequency;

2. Clinical signs were assessed using slit lamp biomicroscopy (Topcon®), as follows:

a) Conjunctival injection, considered non-existent or mild in grade 1, moderate or regional in grade 2, diffuse in grade 3 and severe with episcleral or scleral involvement in grade 4 (MCMONNIES; HO, 2009);

b) Conjunctival colour was assessed using rose bengal 1% and fluorescein sodium 1% (Ophthalmos-Ophthalmos® Indústria e Comércio de Produtos Farmacêuticos LTDA). For this gradation, we preferred to divide the ocular surface into three parts: temporal bulbar conjunctiva, nasal conjunctiva and corneal area, scoring each region from 0 to 3, with "0" being *the* absence of colouring, "1" being light colouring, "2" being diffuse colouring, but not filling the entire area, and "3" being that which fills the entire area. The total results in a maximum of "9", which is why it is suggested to average the 3 areas (PEREIRA GOMES; LIMA; ADAN, 1999; VAN BIJSTERVELD, 1969). So, if the average resulted in a value of "0 to 1", the DEWS grade would be 1, "1 to 2" would be DEWS grade 2, "2 to 3" would be DEWS grade 3, and a score of "3" would be DEWS grade "4".

c) Corneal colour was graded as mentioned above, but the cornea was divided into 3 regions: superior, middle and inferior, and the average of each region was also calculated and graded according to DEWS (VAN BIJSTERVELD, 1969).

d) other signs on the cornea or in the tear film: in grade 1 there are no mild omissions; in grade 2 there is a reduction in the tear meniscus (less than 0.35mmugere echo eye) and an increase in debris; in grade 3 there may be filamentary keratitis in addition to the signs of grade 2; in grade 4 there are all the signs of grade 3 and there may also be corneal ulceration.

e) Alterations to the eyelids and meibomian glands can also appear in grades 1 to 4. They may or may not be present in grades 1 to 2, and are frequent in grade 3, while in grade 4 there is already keratinisation, trichiasis, and even blepharus.

f) TRFL (tear film break up time) or TFBUT (tear film break up time), graded from 1 to 4, where grade 1 means variable or normal tear film break up time, grade 2 means that the BUT is less than or equal to 10 seconds, grade 3 is less than or equal to 5 seconds, and grade 4 is immediate tear film break up. The BUT is carried out by instilling fluorescein and asking the patient to blink, marking how long it takes for the first "defect" or "break" in the tear film to appear (CHO et al., 1998).

g) The Schirmer test is also evaluated in the severity table, grade 1 - its value (in millimetres) is variable or normal, grade 2 is less than or equal to 10mm, grade 3 is less than or equal to 5mm, and in grade 4 it is less than or equal to 2mm. The Schirmer test used was the Schirmer I test, which consists of using standard 5 x 35mm #41 millimetre filter paper (Ophthalmos-Ophthalmos® Indústria e Comércio de Produtos Farmacêuticos LTDA), on the temporal limit of the middle third of the patients' lower eyelids, without the use of anaesthetic, assessing how much the paper is moist after 5 minutes, which reflects tear secretion (VAN BIJSTERVELD, 1969).

h) Visual acuity: using the Snellen chart and recording the best corrected visual acuity of both eyes;

Patients were also assessed using the OSDI (Ocular Surface Disease Index-Allergan) questionnaire, with scores recorded before and after treatment (SCHIFFMAN et al., 2000).

All these patients were also examined for:

Applanation tonometry using a Goldmann tonometer, biomicroscopy (using a Topcon® slit lamp), which assessed other ocular surface and lens alterations in addition to the above signs, fundoscopy (using a Volk® 90DP lens), performed under mydriasis with mydriacyl and 10% phenylephrine (Ophthalmos- Ophthalmos® Indústria e Comércio de Produtos Farmacêuticos LTDA), to detect vitreoretinal or choroidal pathologies, especially diabetic retinopathy. 5.7 Intervention

Clinical assessment: the patients selected for treatment underwent a full blood count, serological tests for Chagas, syphilis, cytomegalovirus, HTLV, HIV and hepatitis B and C. With negative serologies and blood counts within normal parameters, they were referred to the state blood bank (Hemocentro de Alagoas - HEMOAL) and underwent an anamnesis and physical examination with a single haematologist.

Due to the difficulty in gaining peripheral venous access, we chose the autologous donation technique at rather than the platelet apheresis technique, because although the latter produces a higher final number of platelets, it requires the patient to have a minimum blood flow rate for it to work, as well as costing around ten times more than the donation technique.

Patients deemed fit underwent autologous donation by venipuncture of the median vein of the elbow. 350 ml of whole blood was collected in a triple bag previously prepared with SAG mannitol as an anticoagulant and CPD (sodium citrate, phosphate and dextrose) as a preservative. The blood was processed in a refrigerated centrifuge (SORVALL-RC3BP+®), where in the first centrifugation, the plasma was separated from the red blood cells at a frequency of 2000 revolutions for 5 minutes, and in the second centrifugation to separate the plasma from the platelets, the frequency was 3800 revolutions for 10 minutes. The final product, which was the random platelet concentrate, was prepared in a sterile laminar flow room and stored in sterile eye drops of 5 ml each, with calcium gluconate as the vehicle. The eye drops were sent to the Microbiology Service of the CPML (Centre for Medical Laboratory Pathology of the University of Health Sciences of Alagoas (UNCISAL). The blood was cultured for bacteria and fungi on HEMOPROV®-type culture media.

Patients discontinued previous treatment for dry eye 5 days before using CCP. They were instructed to wash their hands before applying the product, to keep the application area clean and not to touch the dropper. The patient was advised to keep the bottle of eye drops in use at +4°C and the rest at -20°C.

Patients were advised to discard the eye drops they were using after 7 days and look for new eye drops to use, frozen at -20 degrees Celsius, which were kept in a specific freezer at the Blood Bank (HEMOAL).

The patient was instructed to use 1 drop every 6 hours in both eyes for 30 days. These patients were examined weekly using biomicroscopy and fundoscopy and after 30 days, a new assessment was carried out using the same tests carried out before treatment, to assess the severity of the dry eye.

5.8 Statistical method

5.8.1 Sample size calculation

The sample size was defined by convenience.

5.8.2 Statistical analysis

The means and standard deviations of the "age" variable were calculated, as well as the median and interquartile range of all the other variables, using Biostat 5.3 software (AYRES et al., [s.d.]).

To analyse the degree of severity before and after treatment, each variable in the DEWS table was assessed using the value for one eye (DRY EYE WORKSHOP, 2007c), the Schirmer test and the TRFL were analysed using the average of the values for both eyes, and visual acuity was calculated using the values for each eye separately, and for symptoms, both eyes were considered mutually.

The Wilcoxon test was used to determine statistical significance, and p-values <0.05 were considered statistically significant. Visual acuity was assessed using the values of both eyes separately.

CHAPTER 6

RESULTS

6.1 The selected patients

A total of 221 diabetic patients were referred to the Ophthalmology department, from which 58 patients were selected who met the criteria for CCP treatment, having moderate to severe symptomatic dry eye (corresponding to one or more symptoms of DEWS severity level 2 to 4, and one or more clinical signs or a positive objective test (Schirmer test less than or equal to 10mm in 5 minutes or TRFL (tear film break-up time) less than 10 seconds).Of the 58, nine were lost to follow-up, with one excluded because of dementia, ten because they were using antiglaucoma eye drops, two because of keratitis and two who died before treatment began. Of the remaining 34 patients, nine were not interested in undergoing treatment, despite their symptoms and clinical signs. The remaining 25 patients were refractory or unresponsive to conventional therapy for dry eye and were selected for treatment with CCP. They underwent an assessment to investigate conditions that would contraindicate autologous donations, and three were excluded because of clinical conditions (one patient with severe heart disease, one with hypertensive crisis, one with a recent stroke, i.e. less than six months old), four because they didn't have venous access available for venepuncture, four were excluded because they tested positive for blood-borne diseases (one with HIV and syphilis, one with HIV, one with Chagas disease and HTLV, and one with hepatitis B), one was excluded because his blood culture for bacteria was positive. One patient abandoned treatment and follow-up (Figure 2).

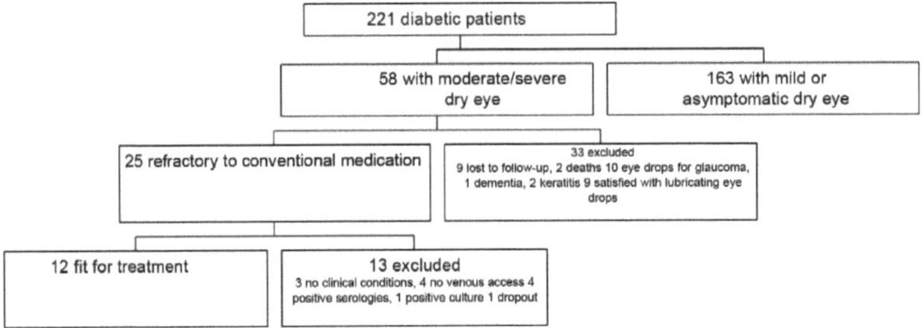

Figure 2: Patient selection flowchart

6.2 The epidemiological profile of patients

Of the 12 patients who underwent CCP treatment and were assessed in this study, 11 were women and 1 was a man. The mean age of the patients was 59.5 ± 11.58 (SD).

Regarding the ethnicity of the selected patients, 04 (33.33%) were white, 06 (50%) brown and 02 (16.67%) black. The average fasting glycaemia of these patients was 195.42 ± 95.95 mg/dl. The average duration of the disease was 11.25 ± 7.04 years.

As for schooling, 01 (8.33%) patient reported not being literate, 01 (8.33%) had completed literacy, 06 (50%) had incomplete first degree, 02 (16.67%) had completed second degree, 01 (8.33%) had incomplete higher education and 01 (8.33%) had completed higher education.

Eleven of the patients were housewives and one was an administrative technician.

With regard to family income, 07 (58.33%) reported receiving one minimum wage, 02 (16.67%) reported receiving two minimum wages, 02 (16.67%) reported receiving between two and four minimum wages. With regard to systemic comorbidities and medication, the results are shown in Table 1.

Table 1. Comorbidities and medication use of the 12 patients treated.

Comorbidity/medications	Prevalence (%)
HAS	50
Asthma	16,67
Osteoarthritis	16,67
Thyroid nodule	8,33
Oral hypoglycaemic agents	100
ARA	25
Diuretics	25
Insulin	16,67
ACEI	16,67
Benzodiazepines	16,67
Proton pump inhibitor	8,33
AAS	8,33
Lipid-lowering agents	8,33
Calcium channel blocker	8,33
Beta-blocker	8,33

Caption: SAH= systemic arterial hypertension, ARA= angiotensin receptor antagonists, ACEI= angiotensin-converting enzyme inhibitors, ASA= acetylsalicylic acid.
Source: author.

With regard to eye diseases and the use of eye drops, the results are described in Table 2.

Table 2. Pathologies, medications and ocular history.

Eye pathology/medications/background	Incidence (%)
Diabetic retinopathy	50
Cataract	16,67
Glaucoma	16,67
Pterygium	8,33
Previous eye surgery	50
Use of lubricants	100
Use of ciclosporin	8,33

Source: author.

6.3 The results of the symptoms

The overall results for the symptoms are compiled in Table 3.

In the evaluation of symptoms, there was a significant improvement in patients treated with

CCP. Complaints of dryness, itching or foreign body sensation, burning, red eye (or hyperaemia), crusts and mucus were considered ocular discomfort.

As for dry eyes, the patients had a median grade of 3 (3-3) before CCP and 1 (1-2) after one month ($p = 0.002$). All patients (12/12) showed a reduction in the severity gradient for this symptom and, of these, 66.67% (8/12) had total improvement of this symptom (grade 1) and 33.33% (4/12) had partial improvement.

For the complaint of foreign body sensation, patients had a median grade of 3 (3-3) before CCP and 1.5 (1-2) after one month ($p = 0.002$). All (12/12) showed a reduction in the severity gradient for this symptom and, of these, 50% (6/12) had a total improvement in this symptom (grade 1) and 50% (6/12) had a partial improvement.

Regarding the symptom of burning, patients had a median grade of 3 (3-3) before CCP, and 1 (1-1) after one month ($p = 0.002$). All (12/12) had total improvement of this symptom (grade 1).

The report of red eyes or hyperaemia among the patients had a median gradation of 3 (2-3) before CCP, and 1 (1-1) after one month ($p = 0.005$). All patients (12/12) showed a reduction in the severity gradient for this symptom, 91.67% (11/12) had a total improvement in this symptom (grade 1) and 8.33% (1/12) had a partial improvement.

With regard to complaints of crusts and mucus, the patients had a median grade of 1 (1-1) before CCP, and 1 (1-1) one month after ($p = 0.17$), but only 16.67% (2/12) had these symptoms before treatment, so both patients showed total improvement (grade 1) of their symptoms.

After ocular discomfort, the other item in the severity classification was the complaint of blurred vision. Patients had a median gradation of 2 (1.75-3) before CCP, and 2 (1-2) after one month ($p = 0.018$), 58.33% (7/12) showed a decrease in the severity gradation for this symptom. However, only 75% (9/12) had this symptom before CCP, so 77.78% (7/9) showed a decrease in severity, and of these, 2 of the 9 showed total improvement (grade 1) of their symptoms.

6.4 Clinical signs

After the topics of symptoms - ocular discomfort - and the report of blurred vision, the results of the clinical signs and objective tests were then recorded, still according to the table at severity classification of DEWS.

The following signs are summarised in Table 4 and some are illustrated in the photos below.

Table 3: Dry eye symptoms characterising ocular discomfort according to DEWS criteria

	Dry eyes		Feeling of sand		Eye burning		Red eyes		Crusty eyelashes/sticky eyes in the morning		Visual clouding	
	Before	After 1 month	Befor e	After 1 month	Before	After 1 month	Before	After 1 month	Before	Afte r 1 month	Befor e	After 1 month
Patient 1	3	2	3	2	3	1	1	1	1	1	1	1
Patient 2	3	1	3	1	3	1	3	1	1	1	3	2
Patient 3	3	1	3	1	3	1	3	1	1	1	3	2
Patient 4	3	1	3	2	3	1	3	1	1	1	2	2
Patient 5	3	1	3	1	3	1	3	1	3	1	3	2
Patient 6	4	1	4	2	4	1	4	1	4	1	4	3
Patient 7	3	2	3	2	3	1	3	2	1	1	3	2
Patient 8	3	1	3	1	3	1	2	1	1	1	2	1
Patient 9	3	1	3	1	3	1	2	1	1	1	1	1
Patient 10	3	2	3	2	3	1	3	1	1	1	2	2
Patient 11	3	1	3	1	3	1	2	1	1	1	1	1
Patient 12	3	2	3	2	3	1	1	1	1	1	2	1
	p=0,002		p=0,002		p=0,002		p=0,005		p=0,17		p=0,018	

Key: 1: never, 2: infrequently, 3: frequently, 4: constantly
Source: author

With regard to the clinical sign of conjunctival injection, the patients had a median gradation of 1(1-2) before CCP and 1(1-1) after CCP (p=0.07). Of the 12 patients, 33.33% had a decrease in the gradation of hyperaemia severity (4/12), and 66.67% remained unchanged. However, only 4 had hyperaemia before and, of these, 3 had total improvement (grade 1).

As for conjunctival colouration, the patients had a median gradation of 1.5(1-2) before CCP, and 1(1-2) after CCP (p=0.03). Of the 12 patients, 50% had improved colour (6/12), and 50% remained unchanged. However, only 6 had staining before and all of this (100%) had total improvement (grade 1).

Regarding corneal colouring, the patients had a median gradation of 1(1-1) before CCP and 1(1-1) after CCP (p=0.18). Of the 12 patients, only 2 had some corneal staining before and, of these, both had a reduction in the severity gradient, but only one of the two had a total improvement in this sign (grade 1).

Patient 6 - Fluorescein staining before and after CCP treatment.

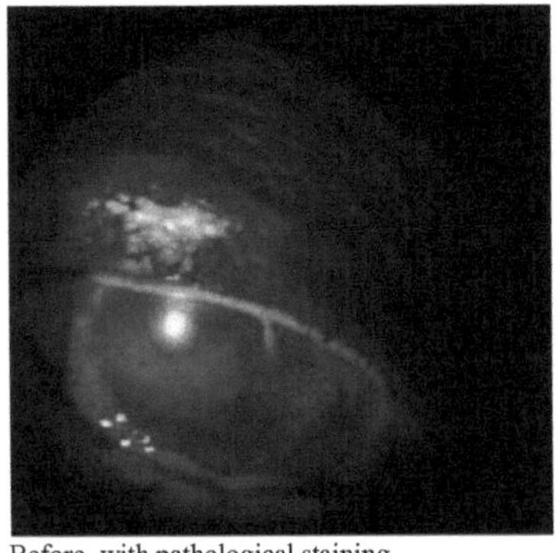

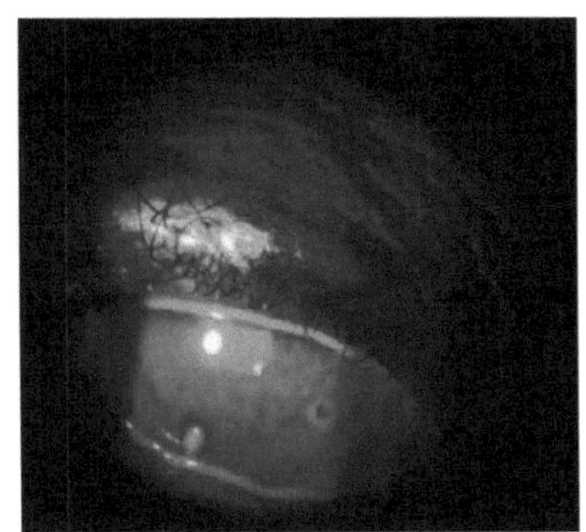

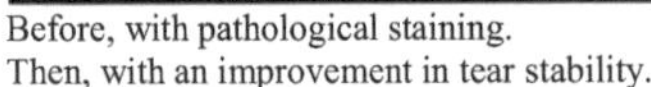

Before, with pathological staining.
Then, with an improvement in tear stability.

Patient 8 - Fluorescein staining before and after CCP treatment.

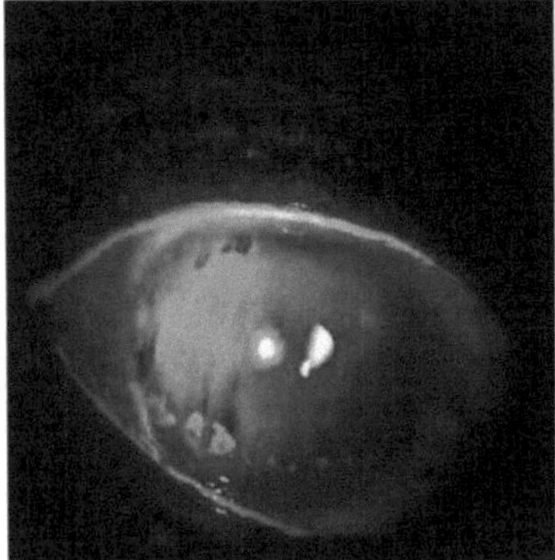

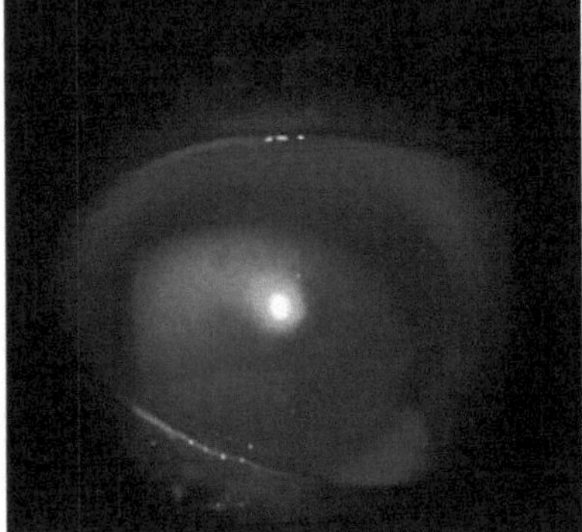

Before, with pathological colouring.
Then, with an improvement in tear stability.

As for other tear and corneal signs, such as the evaluation of the lacrimal meniscus, the patients had a median grade of 2(2-2) before CCP, and 1(1-1.25) after CCP ($p=0.005$). Of the 12 patients, 83.33% had a reduction in the severity of these signs (10/12), of these 9 out of 12 had total improvement (grade 1) and 16.67% (2/12) remained with the same alterations.

Patient 1 - Lacrimal meniscus before and after CCP treatment

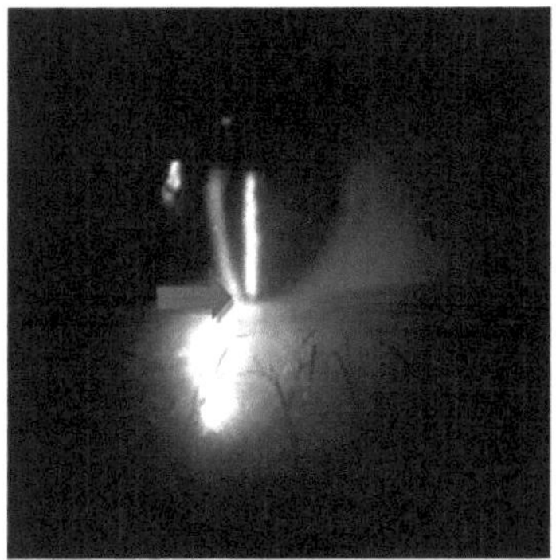

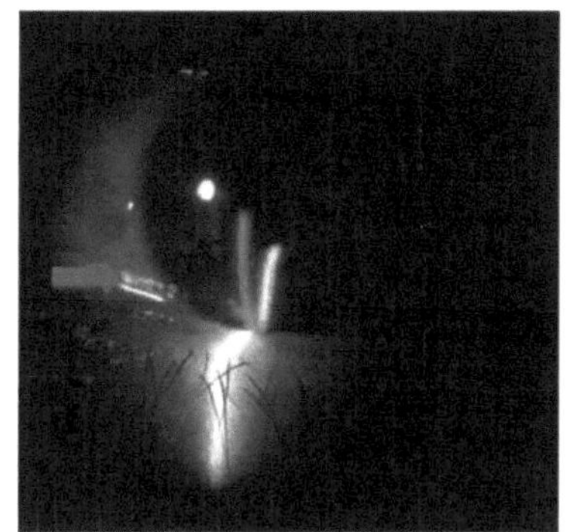

Before, almost inevitable.
Then it became more obvious.

Patient 2 - Lacrimal meniscus before and after CCP treatment.

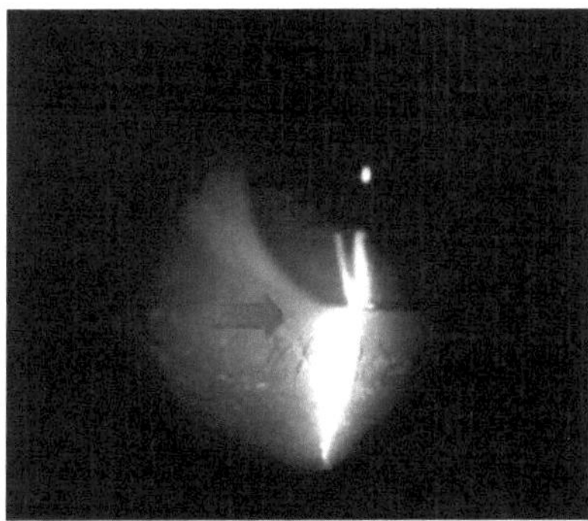

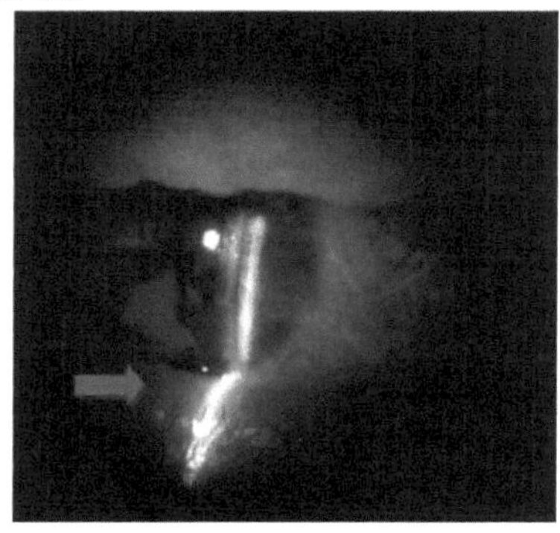

Before, almost inevitable.
Then it became more obvious.

Patient 3 - Lacrimal meniscus before and after CCP treatment.

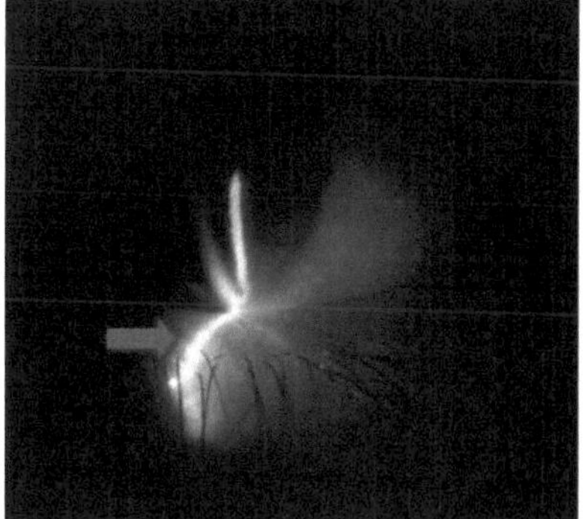

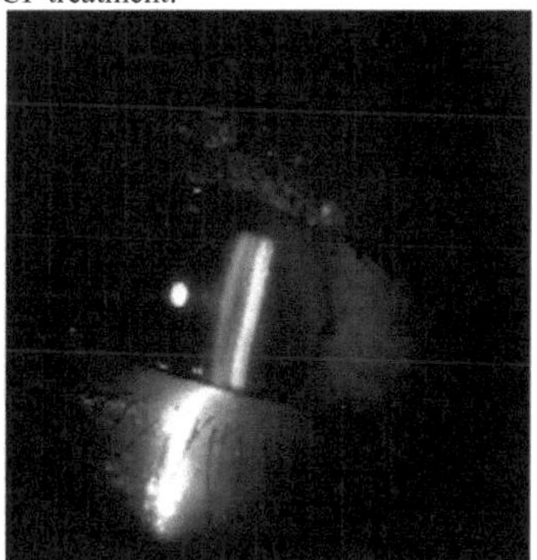

Before, almost inevitable.
Then it became more obvious.

Patient 4 - Lacrimal meniscus before and after CCP treatment.

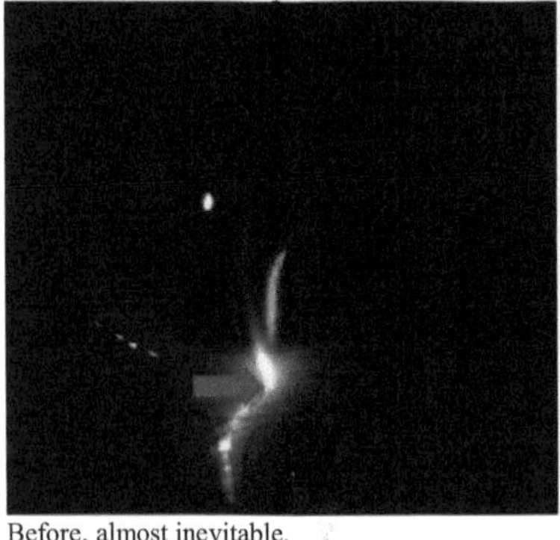

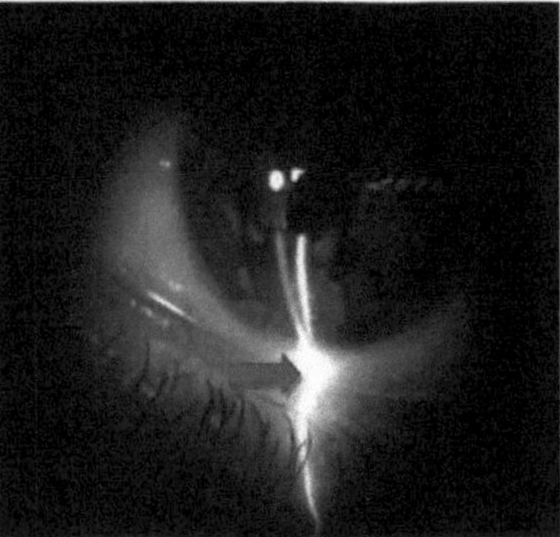

Before, almost inevitable.
Then it became more obvious.

Patient 5 - Lacrimal meniscus before and after CCP treatment.

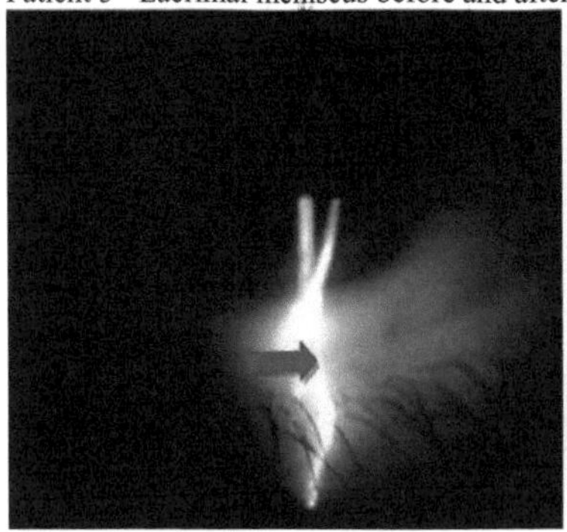

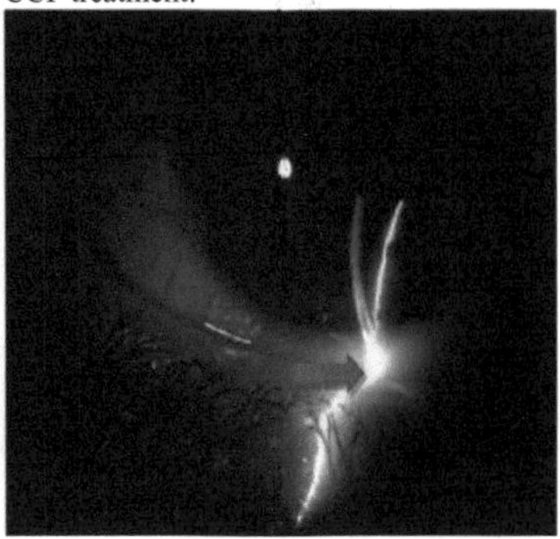

Before, almost inevitable.
Then it became more obvious.

Patient 6 - Lacrimal meniscus before and after CCP treatment.

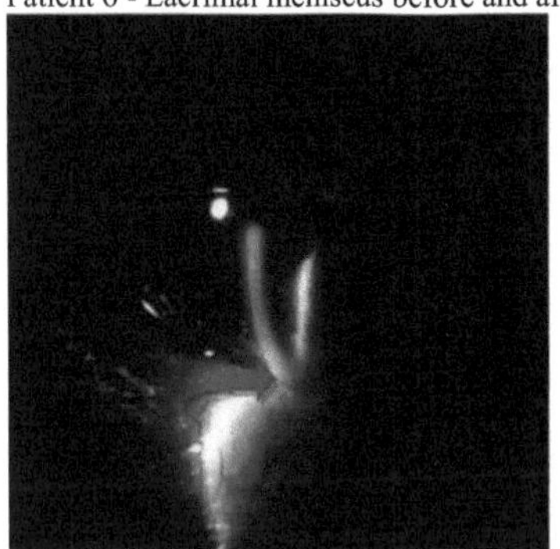

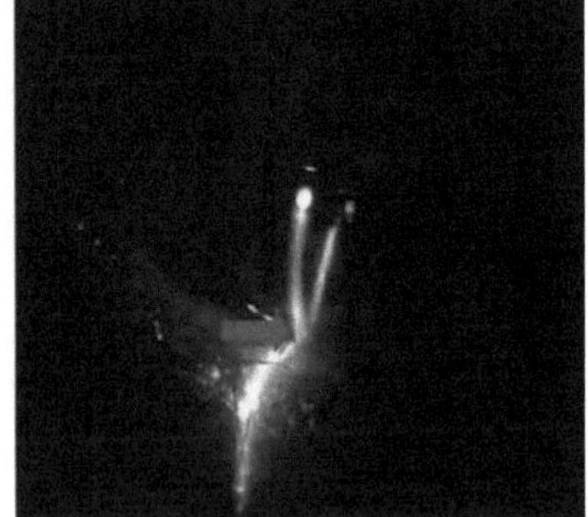

Before, almost inevitable.
Then it became more obvious.

Patient 7 - Lacrimal meniscus before and after CCP treatment.

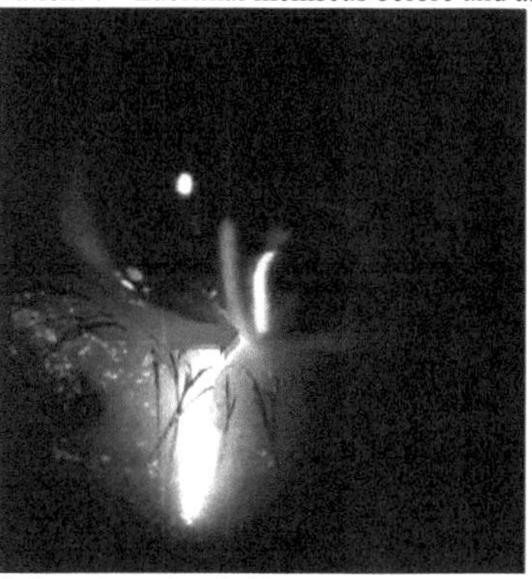

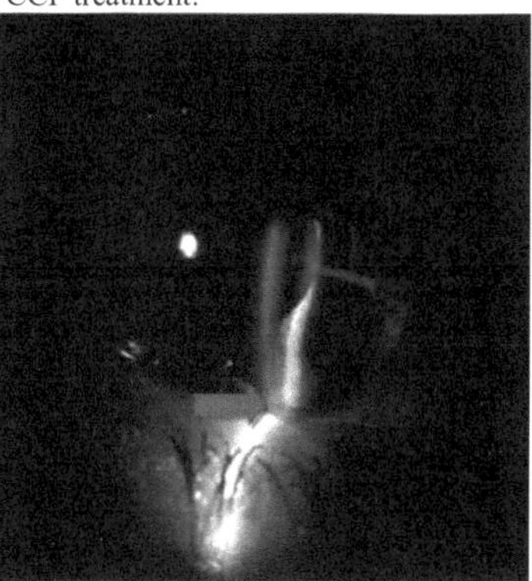

Before, almost inevitable.
Then it became more obvious.

Patient 8 - Lacrimal meniscus before and after CCP treatment.

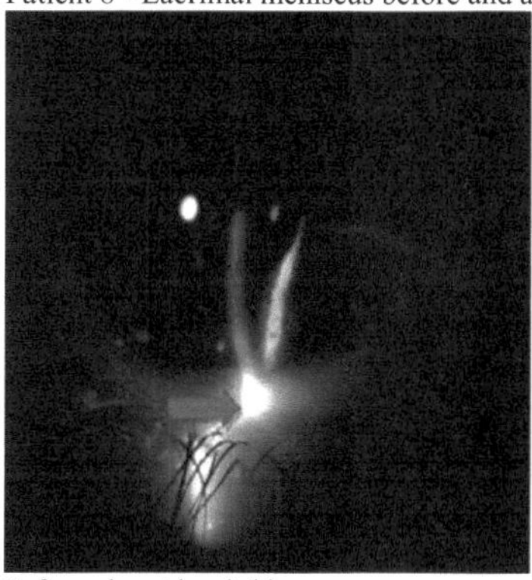

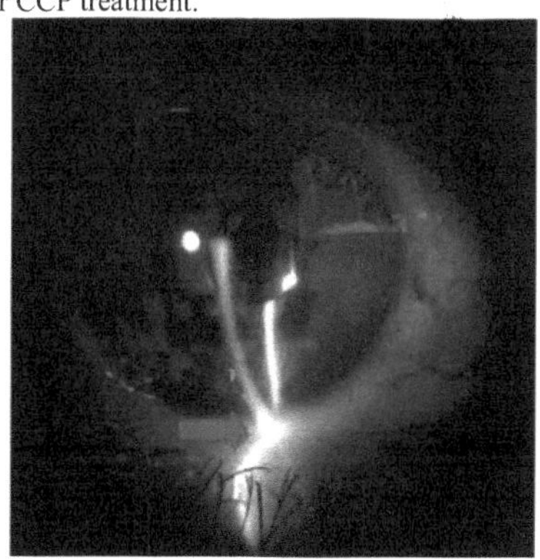

Before, almost inevitable.
Then it became more obvious.

Patient 9 - Lacrimal meniscus before and after CCP treatment.

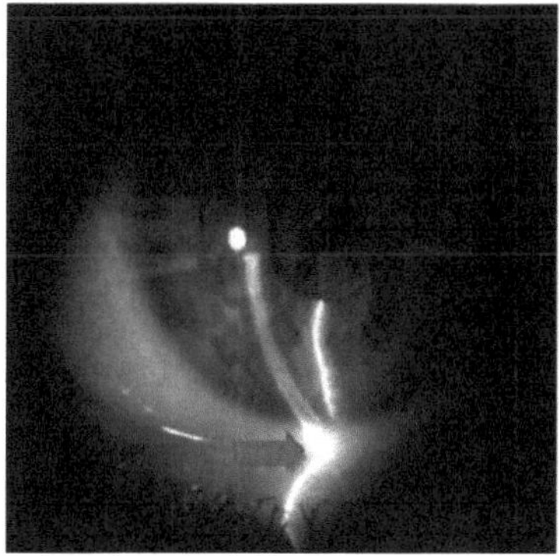

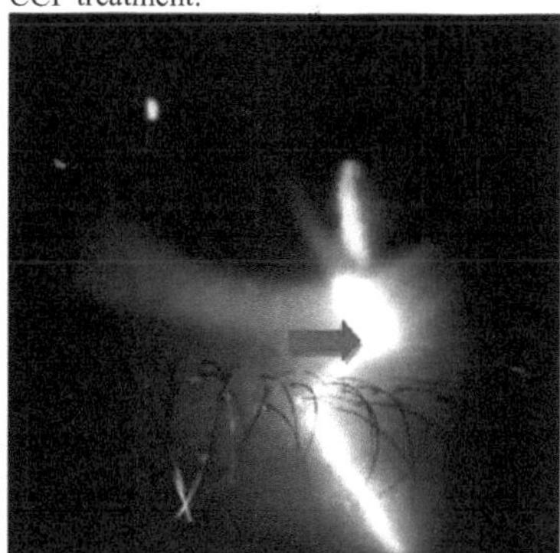

Before, almost inevitable.
Then it became more obvious.

Patient 10 - Lacrimal meniscus before and after CCP.

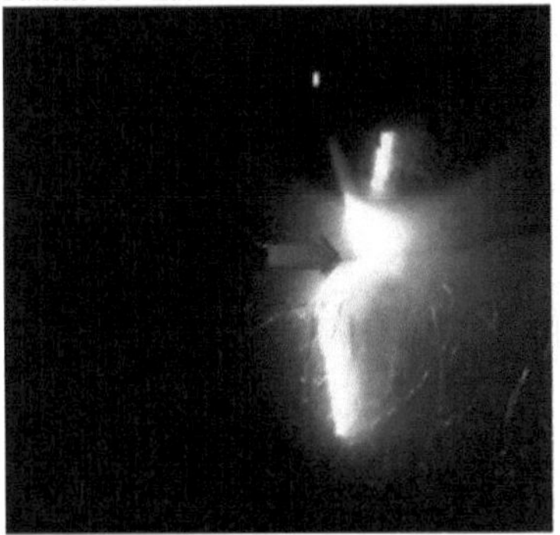

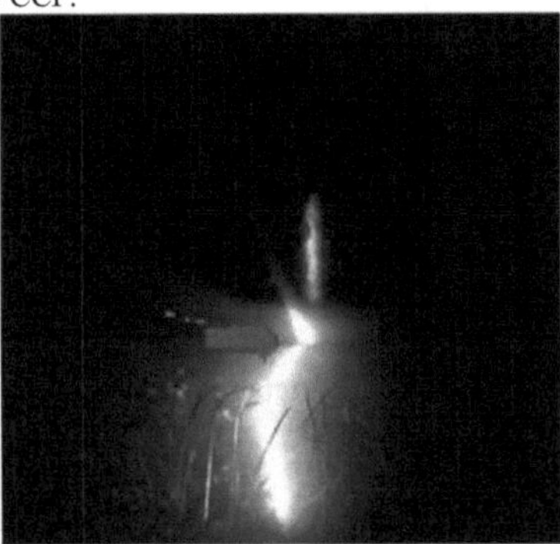

Before, almost inevitable.
Then it became more obvious.

Patient 11 - Lacrimal meniscus before and after CCP treatment.

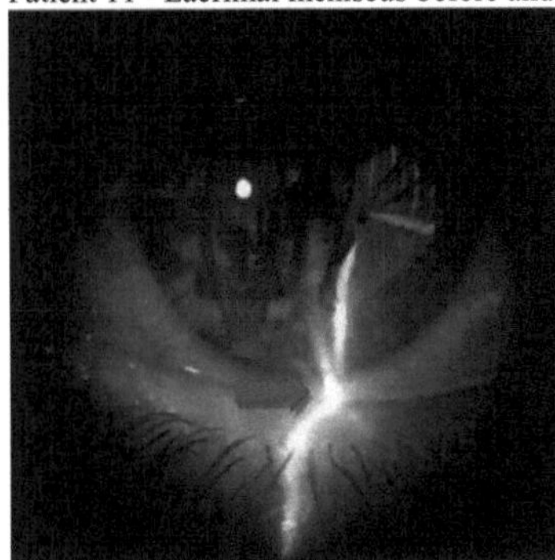

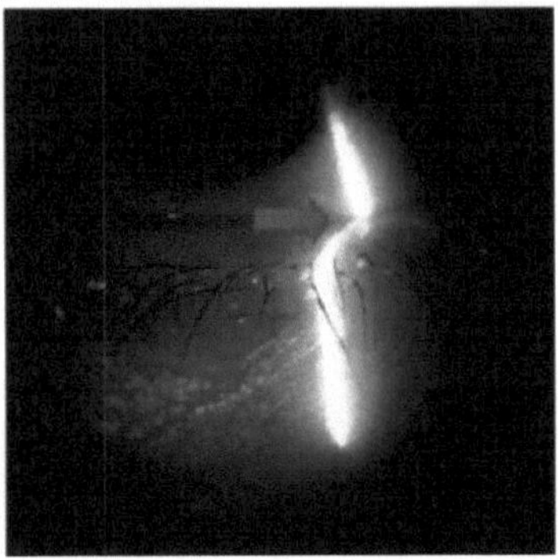

Before, almost inevitable.
Then it became more obvious.

Patient 12 - Lacrimal meniscus before and after CCP treatment.

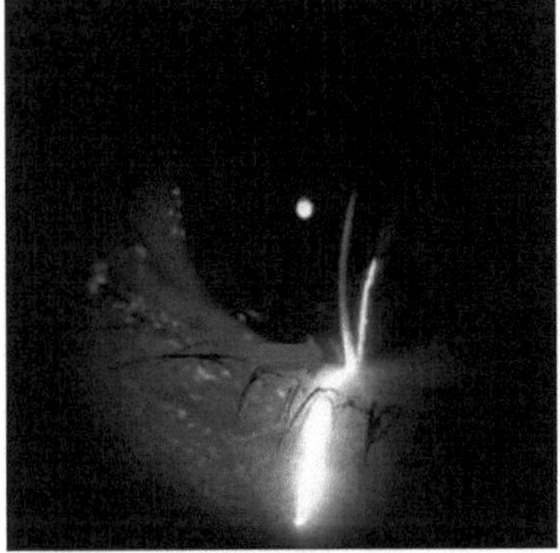

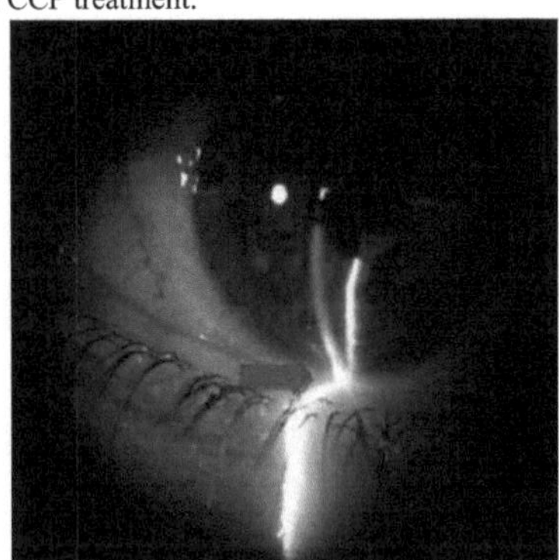

Before, almost inevitable.
Then it became more obvious.

Meibomius gland dysfunction and eyelid changes were also assessed. Patients had a median gradation of 1(1-1.5) before CCP and 1(1-1) after CCP (p=0.18). Of the 12 patients, 16.67% had an improvement in these alterations and (1/12) or 8.33% remained in the same situation. Therefore, only 3 had alterations before, and of these, 66.67% (2/3) had total improvement (grade 1) of this sign.

Table 4 Clinical signs of dry eye according to DEWS criteria

	Hyperaemia		Conjunctival colouring		Corneal colouring		Corneal and tear signs		Changes in the eyelids and glands	
	Before	After 1 month	Before	After 1 month	Before	After 1 month	Before	After 1 month	Before	After 1 month
Patient 1	1	1	1	1	1	1	2	1	1	1
Patient 2	1	1	1	1	1	1	2	1	3	1
Patient 3	1	1	1	1	1	1	2	1	1	1
Patient 4	1	1	2	1	1	1	2	1	1	1
Patient 5	1	1	1	1	1	1	2	1	1	1
Patient 6	3	2	3	1	4	3	3	2	4	4
Patient 7	1	1	2	1	1	1	2	1	1	1
Patient 8	1	1	2	1	2	1	2	1	3	1
Patient 9	1	1	1	1	1	1	2	2	1	1
Patient 10	2	1	1	1	1	1	2	1	1	1
Patient 11	2	1	2	1	1	1	2	1	1	1
Patient 12	2	1	2	1	1	1	2	2	1	1
	p=0,07		p=0,03		p=0,18		p=0,005		p=0,18	

Legend Conjunctival Hyperaemia and Colouring 1: absent, 2: mild, 3: moderate, 4: significant or severe
Legend Corneal staining 1: absent, 2: mild, 3: moderate predominantly central, 4: significant or severe (diffuse)
Legend Corneal and tear signs 1: Absent, 2: Decreased tear meniscus and debris in the tear, 3: Presence of mucus or filament, 4: Filamentary keratitis, mucus and possible corneal ulcer
Legend Eyelid and gland changes 1: absent, 2: mild meibomitis, 3: moderate blepharitis, 4: trichiasis, symblepharitis, scarring
Source: author

6.5 . The objective tests

The Schirmer I and TRFL tests are summarised in Table 5.

As for the Schirmer test, the mean values between both eyes were used. Considering the gradation value in the Schirmer test (from 1 to 4 as mentioned in the methods), the patients had a median gradation of 3 (2-3) before CCP, and 2 (1-3) after one month of treatment (p = 0.11). Among the 12 patients, 41.67% (5/12) had a decrease in the severity gradient of the test, 50% (6/12) had no change in this gradient and 8.33% (1/12) had a reduced value in the test after treatment.

However, considering the raw value in millimetres of the Schirmer test, using the average between the two eyes, the median was 5 (4-9.25) before CCP, and 8 (5-12.25) after treatment. The mean was 6.75mm ± 3.66 before and 8.96mm ± 4.56 after treatment (P = 0.04). On this basis, 66.67% (8/12) showed an improvement in this test, 25% (3/12) had no change and 1 patient (8.33%) evolved with a lower test value after treatment.

The tear film break-up time (TRFL) test had a median gradation of 2.5 (2-3) before CCP, and 2 (1.75-3) after one month (p = 0.018). Among the twelve patients, 58.33% (7/12) had a decrease in the severity gradient of the test and 41.66% (12/05) had no change in this gradient, some findings of which are recorded in the following images.

Patient 1 - Fluorescein staining (tear film stability-TRFL) before and after CCP treatment.

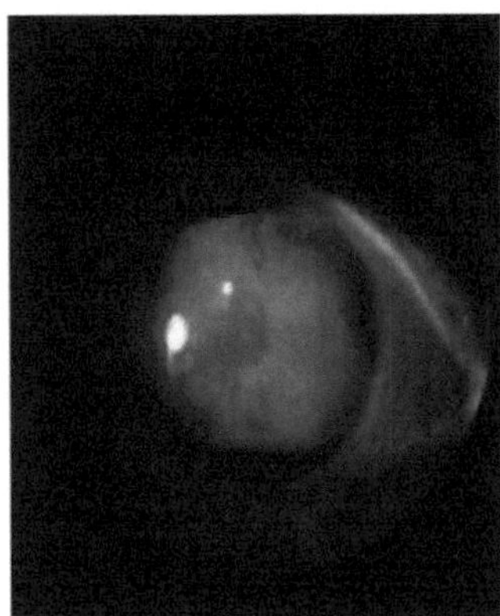

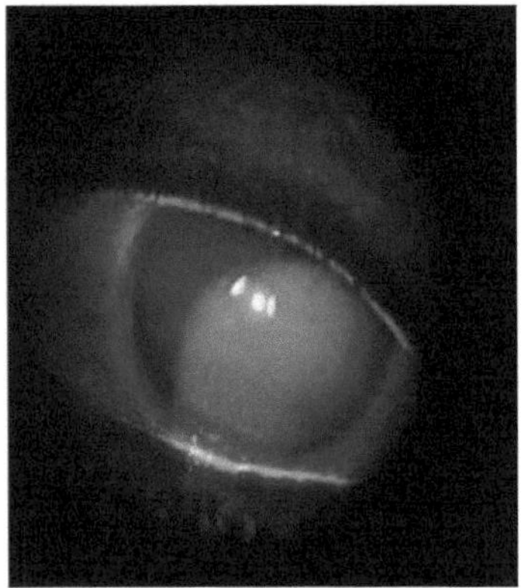

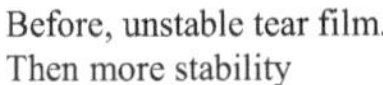

Before, unstable tear film.
Then more stability

Patient 2 - Fluorescein staining (tear film stability-TRFL) before and after CCP treatment.

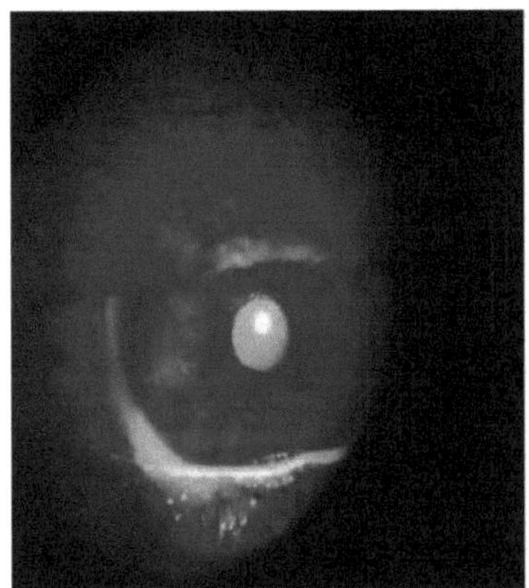

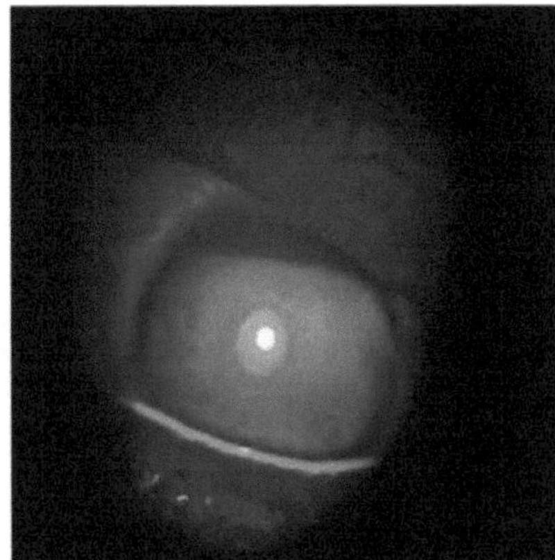

Before, unstable tear film.
Then more stability.

Patient 3 - Fluorescein staining (tear film stability-TRFL) before and after CCP treatment.

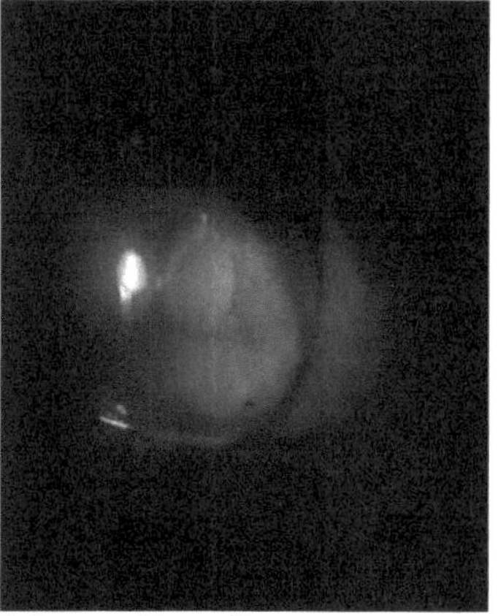

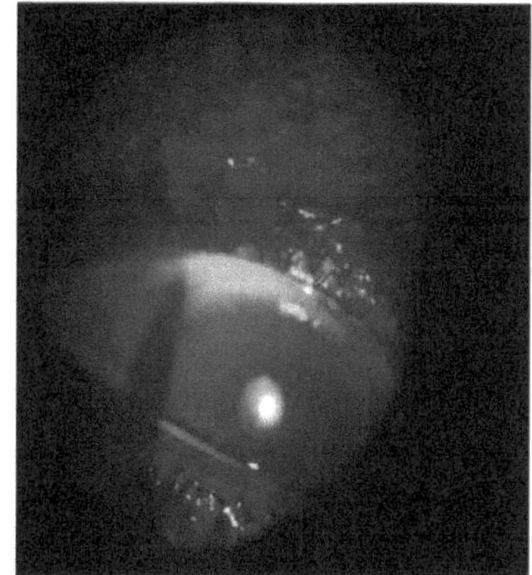

Before, unstable tear film.
Then more stability.

Patient 4 - Fluorescein staining (tear film stability-TRFL) before and after CCP treatment.

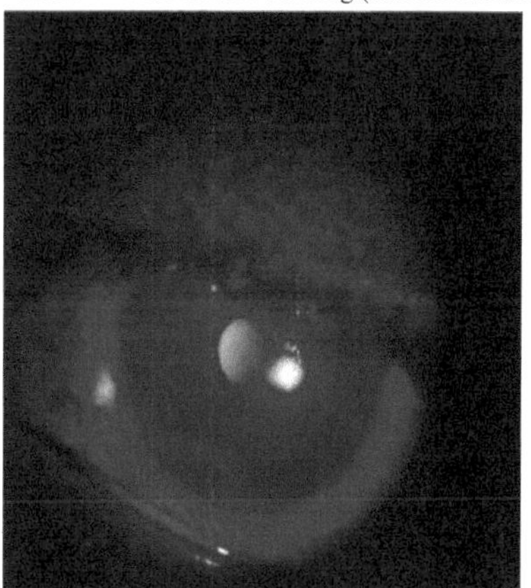

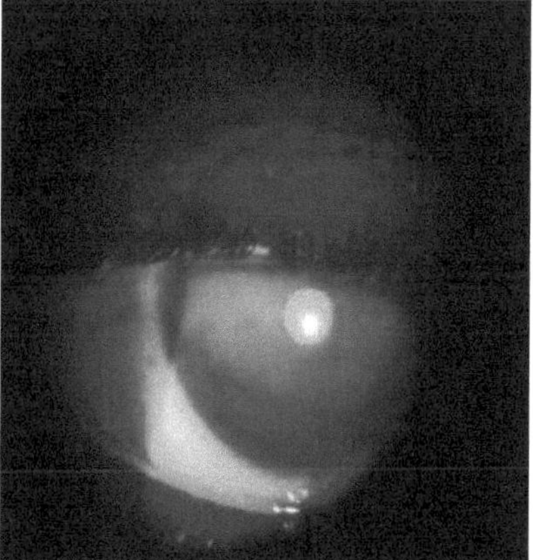

Before, unstable tear film.
Then more stability.

Patient 5 - Fluorescein staining (tear film stability-TRFL) before and after CCP treatment.

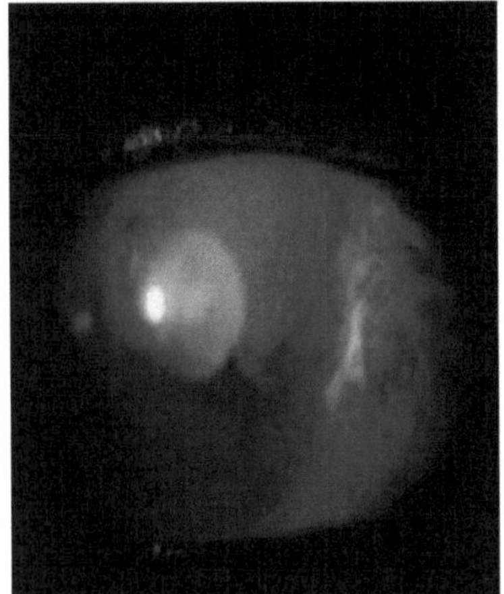

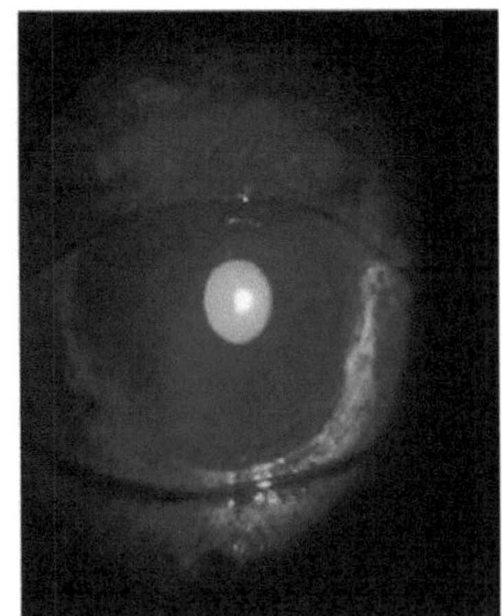

Before, unstable tear film.
Then more stability.

Patient 7 - Fluorescein staining (tear film stability -TRFL) before and after CCP treatment.

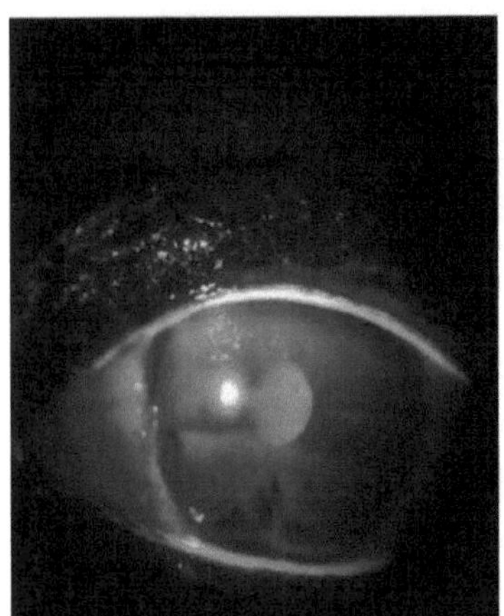

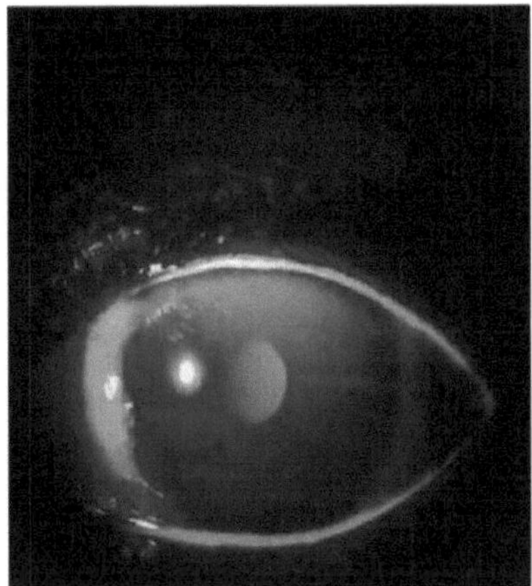

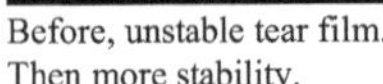

Before, unstable tear film.
Then more stability.

Patient 9 - Fluorescein staining (tear film stability -TRFL) before and after CCP treatment.

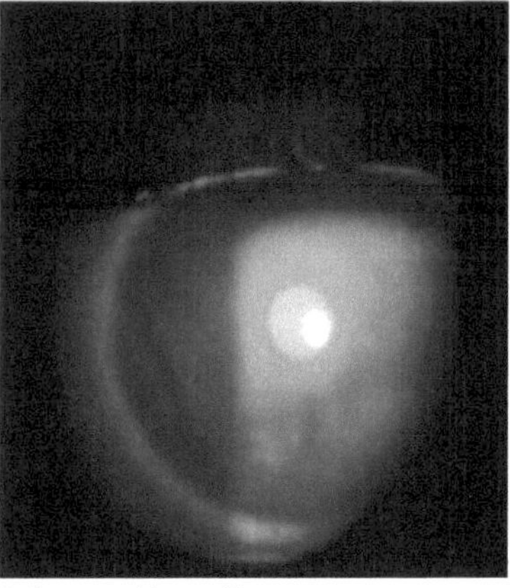

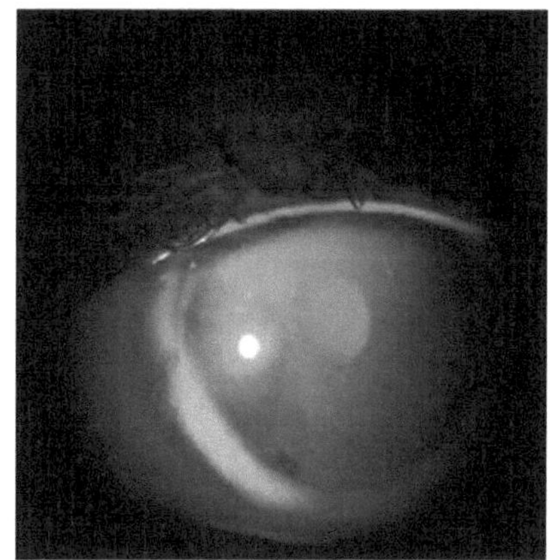

Before, unstable tear film.
Then more stability.

Patient 10 - Fluorescein staining (tear film stability -TRFL) before and after CCP treatment.

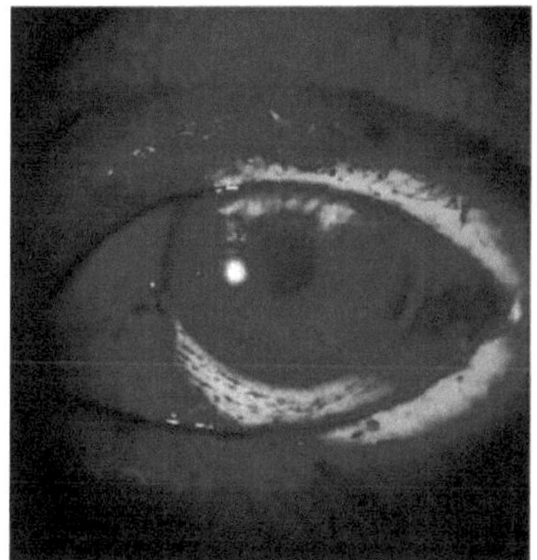

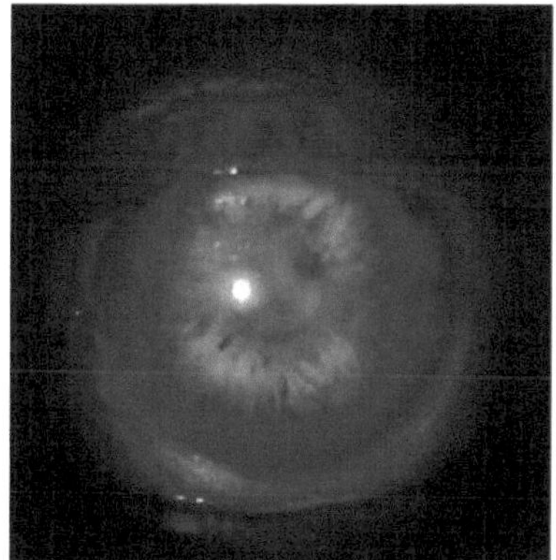

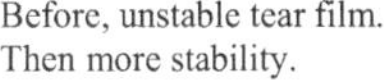

Before, unstable tear film.
Then more stability.

Patient 11 - Fluorescein staining (tear film stability-TRFL) before and after CCP treatment.

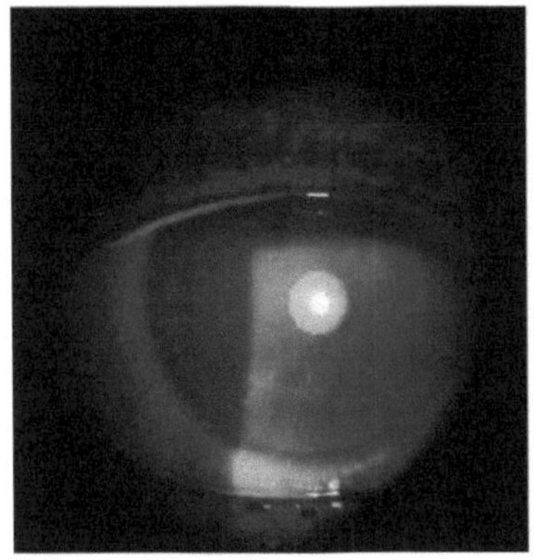

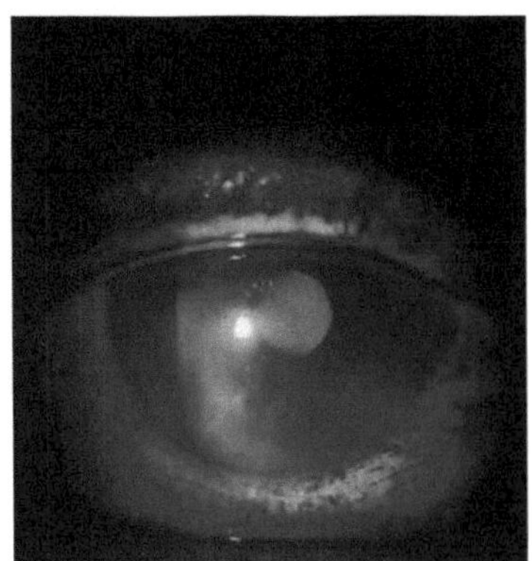

Before, unstable tear film.
Then more stability.

Patient 12 - Fluorescein staining (tear film stability-TRFL) before and after CCP treatment.

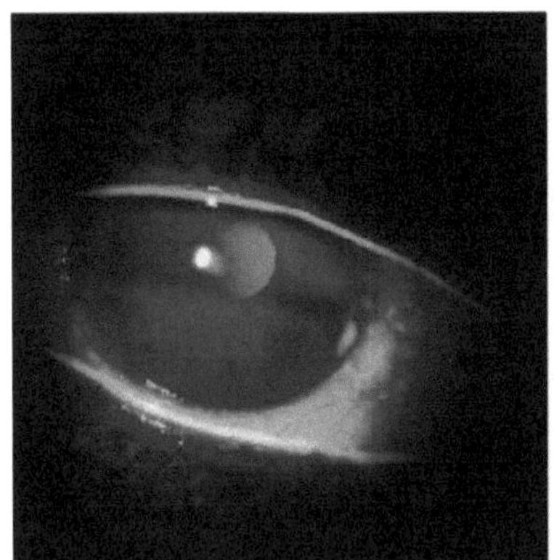

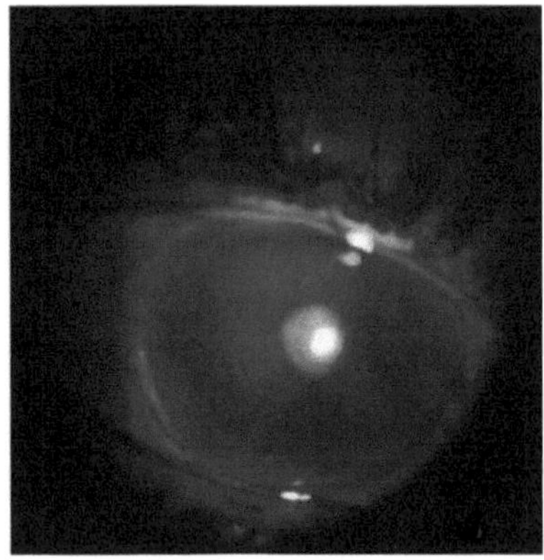

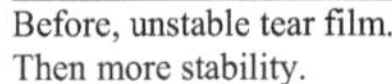

Before, unstable tear film.
Then more stability.

Table 5: Objective tests: severity gradation based on DEWS.

	Schirmer test		BUT or (TRFL)	
	Before	After 1 month	Before	After 1 month
Patient 1	2	3	2	2
Patient 2	4	1	2	2
Patient 3	3	2	2	1
Patient 4	3	3	2	2
Patient 5	2	2	2	1
Patient 6	3	2	3	2
Patient 7	1	1	2	1
Patient 8	3	2	2	1
Patient 9	1	1	2	1
Patient 10	3	3	2	2
Patient 11	2	1	2	1
Patient 12	3	3	2	2
	p=0.ll		p=0,018	

Legend: Schirmer 1: variable schirmer test (greater than or equal to 15mm="normal"); 2: schirmer test less than or equal to lOmm; 3: schirmer test less than or equal to 5mm; 4: schirmer test less than or equal to 2mm
Legend BUT: break up time, 1: variable or greater than 10 seconds (i.e. "normal"); 2: less than or equal to 10 seconds; 3: less than or equal to 5 seconds; 4: immediate
TRFL: tear film break-up time
Source: author

6.6 Visual acuity

Visual acuity was also assessed in a complementary way, but not for classification. Considering the improvement in the number of lines of visual acuity in the right eye, 41.66% (5/12) of the patients had an improvement of one or more lines, 8.33% (1/12) had a reduction of at least one line and 50% (6/12) had no change in acuity in the right eye.

With regard to the improvement in the number of lines of visual acuity in the left eye, 41.66 per cent (5/12) had an improvement of one or more lines and 58.33 per cent (7/12) had no change in the acuity of the left eye.

6.7 The OSDI questionnaire score

The 12 patients were given the OSDI questionnaire before and after using the CCP. The questionnaire is based on the following scores: 0 to 12 considered normal, 13 to 22 mild dry eye, 23 to 32 moderate dry eye and 33 to 100 severe dry eye (SCHIFFMAN et al., 2000).

All the patients (100 per cent) had improved indices after treatment (p=0.002). Evaluating this index alone, before CCP, 11 patients out of 12 (91.67%) had severe dry eye and only 1 (8.33%) had moderate dry eye.

After treatment, 6 of the 12 patients (50%) had indices assessed as normal, 25% (3/12) had dry eye classified as mild, 2 (16.66%) had moderate dry eye and 1 (8.33%) still had severe dry eye. The median score before was 52.4 (48.12-59.67), which dropped to 11.25 (4.32-18.75) after treatment. The mean score before was 56.13±20.94 and after was 13.15±11.40 (Table 6).

6.8 The final DEWS severity classification

Considering the DEWS classification (from 1 to 4), patients presented themselves before and after treatment according to Table 6.

Patients had a median gradation of 3 (2-3) before CCP and 2 (1-2) after one month of treatment ($p = 0.005$). Of the 12 patients, 83.33% obtained some improvement in the severity of dry eye, while 16.67% (2/12) remained with the same gradation.

All patients used the treatment for one month and there were no cases of intolerance or undesirable effects that could be attributed to the use of CCP.

Table 6. Final classification of dry eye severity

	OSDI Score		Degree of Severity DEWS	
	Before	After 1 month	Before	After 1 month
Patient 1	42,5	12,5	2	2
Patient 2	50	10	3	2
Patient 3	32,5	0	3	2
Patient 4	63,8	8,33	3	2
Patient 5	58,3	27,7	2	2
Patient 6	100	15,6	4	3
Patient 7	90	5	2	1
Patient 8	50	22,5	3	1
Patient 9	27,2	0	2	1
Patient 10	54,5	2,27	3	2
Patient 11	52,3	36,4	2	1
Patient 12	52,5	17,5	3	2
	p=0,002		p=0,005	

OSDI legend: 0 to 12: normal eye; 13 to 22: mild dry eye; 23 to 32: moderate dry eye; 33 to 100: severe dry eye
DEWS subtitle: A symptom and a sign at the highest level already characterise the same thing

Source: author

CHAPTER 7

DISCUSSION

Diabetes is one of the main causes of blindness worldwide, and dry eye is one of the ocular alterations that can contribute to this condition. Diabetic patients with dry eye can develop keratopathy, neurotrophic ulcers, corneal opacities, perforation and even loss of vision (MANAVIAT et al., 2008).

The prevalence of dry eye in diabetes has varied between 14 and 54 per cent (CAFFERY et al., 1998)(SHIMMURA; SHIMAZAKI; TSUBOTA, 1999; MOSS; KLEIN; KLEIN, 2000; SCHEIN et al., 1997). This data is compatible with our study, which showed a frequency of 26.2 per cent among the 221 diabetics assessed. The highest incidence of dry eye in general is in females and especially in elderly women, probably due to the decrease in androgen levels at this stage of life, which causes changes in the Meibomius glands (SULLIVAN et al., 2009). Sendecka et al. found an 80 per cent prevalence of dry eye in females over the age of 50, which corroborates our study, in which 11 of the 12 patients were women (SENDECKA; BARYLUK; POLZ-DACEWICZ, 2004). Moss et al, in a 5-year study, observed that the incidence of dry eye increased with age, and in our study, the patients had an average age of over 59 years.

Some studies have shown no predilection between ethnic groups when it comes to dry eye in general (MISRA et al., 2014; SCHAUMBERG et al., 2009). Another study carried out in Scotland, evaluating four groups, Chinese, Indians, Africans and Caucasians, showed lower tear film stability in Chinese, followed by Africans, and better tear film stability in Caucasians (MISRA et al., 2014). It is known that ethnic classification in general is difficult, arbitrary and imperfect (CAVALLI-SFORZA, 2003), which is why there are variables in the literature regarding ethnic classifications, which differ according to the time and reason for the studies. So, based on this information, we prefer to divide our study group into whites, browns (which would include mestizos) and blacks. In the north-east of Brazil, the 2010 census shows that 50.7 per cent of the population are black and mixed-race, which is in line with our findings (IBGE, 2015).

From an epidemiological point of view, the literature found no risk factors such as education or socioeconomic status that could influence dry eye, and a study in Indonesia also showed that profession was not a significant risk factor (SMITH, 2007; LEE et al., 2002). The patients in this study had a relatively low level of education, including the fact that most of them had not completed primary school (66.67%).

Our patients also had a low family income, with 75 per cent earning up to two minimum wages. This didn't interfere with our study either, as they didn't have to pay any costs during this treatment.

With regard to the risk factors for diabetic dry eye, some studies have shown, for example, that dry eye is more frequent in patients with inadequate glycaemic control, mainly occurring during phases of hyperglycaemia due to extracellular hyperosmolarity which affects tear production (NEPP et al., 2000; BINDER et al., 1989; KAISERMAN et al., 2005; SEIFART; STREMPEL, 1994). In our study, fasting glycaemia averaged 195.42± 95.95 mg/dl among the twelve patients selected for treatment, which can be considered high glycaemia (AMERICAN DIABETES ASSOCIATION, 2015).

The average duration of the disease in this study was 11.25 ± 7.04 years. The average found was 25.8 ± 11.4 years in one of the most recent studies in the literature on the epidemiological profile of diabetic dry eye (MISRA et al., 2014). This disparity could be attributed to the socio-economic conditions of these patients, since most of them come from a low social class, including 9 of the 12 who do not have health insurance and use the Unified Health System (SUS), where access to tests takes longer, delaying diagnosis.

Other possible risk factors were the presence of certain comorbidities and the use of certain medications. The analysis of these factors varies greatly in the literature, and a study on the epidemiology of dry eye, carried out by the DEWS subcommittee, listed some factors as relevant and others as uncertain or inconclusive (SMITH, 2007). In our study, 50 per cent of the patients had hypertension (6/12). Schaumberg et al found that the relationship between hypertension and the use of antihypertensive drugs with dry eye was statistically significant (SCHAUMBERG et al., 2009). In a 2000 study, Moss also found a significant relationship between hypertension, allergies and the use of diuretics with dry eye. In 2004, the same author found no relevant results for the association between hypertension, thyroid disease, allergies, among others, and dry eye (MOSS; KLEIN; KLEIN, 2004; MOSS; KLEIN; KLEIN, 2000).

Because of this controversy, we didn't exclude patients with hypertension or those taking medication, since diabetic patients generally use several medications, and we know that these can have different adverse effects from person to person. All of our patients were taking oral hypoglycaemic agents and 2 patients (16.67%) were using insulin. Among the most commonly mentioned antihypertensive drugs were diuretics and angiotensinogen converting enzyme inhibitors. One study showed that the latter medication even played a protective role in the development of dry eye (MOSS; KLEIN; KLEIN, 2004; MOSS; KLEIN; KLEIN, 2000).

With regard to associated ocular pathologies, it was observed that 50% of the patients had diabetic retinopathy, which is compatible with some of the studies on the prevalence of dry eye in diabetes, such as that by Manaviat et al. which showed an incidence of approximately 70% of retinopathy in these patients (MANAVIAT et al., 2008; NAJAFI et al., 2013).

Of the 12 patients, two had cataracts and two had glaucoma, which are some of the ocular manifestations in diabetes (NEGI; VERNON, 2003); 50 per cent had undergone ocular surgery, mainly phacectomy. However, Moss, in his study, found no relationship between cataract surgery or cataract with dry eye (MOSS; KLEIN; KLEIN, 2000), while Yao et al. observed that facectomy can alter the ocular surface and contribute to dry eye (YAO et al., 2015); and the 6 patients who had undergone facectomy in our study did not show severity of dry eye that differed greatly from the others who had not previously undergone surgery.

Because the literature shows that antiglaucoma eye drops can cause ocular surface alterations, such as dry eye, which we have also observed in clinical practice, patients using these drugs were excluded (GOMES et al., 2013).

With regard to the diagnosis of dry eye, it is known that, as it is a multifactorial disease, it is controversial, as the symptoms generally do not correlate with the signs or clinical tests (VERSURA; PROFAZIO; CAMPOS, 2010), and there are numerous ways of classifying, diagnosing and assessing dry eye, which differ widely in the world consensus (BEHRENS et al., 2006), as specialists often use their clinical experience and what is available to them in daily practice.

Diabetes mellitus is known to be an important cause of dry eye, with dysfunctions in both tear quantity and quality, all of which can lead to severe ocular surface alterations such as epithelial fragility, punctate keratopathy, persistent epithelial defects and decreased corneal sensitivity. The end result is irreversible complications such as chronic ocular discomfort, interfering with the patient's quality of life, or visual loss. All of our patients complained of chronic discomfort and reported interference with daily activities (MISRA et al., 2014).

The DEWS recommends obtaining one or more typical symptoms of dry eye and one or more tests. The most commonly used are staining with vital dyes, the Schirmer test and the positive TRFL, which we followed in our study (DRY EYE WORKSHOP, 2007c).

Diagnostic tests for dry eye are therefore of little specificity when used alone, without any combination. Our main criterion for diagnosing and at the same time classifying dry eye was to follow the DEWS severity classification (DRY EYE WORKSHOP, 2007c), which is based on signs and symptoms graded from 1 to 4, where just one symptom associated with any of the positive clinical signs of one of the gradings already configures it.

In one of the few studies evaluating diagnostic tests in diabetic patients specifically, the best diagnostic tests were those with the best sensitivity, specificity and accuracy, with OSDI, TRFL, Schirmer's test, fluorescein staining and tear osmolarity standing out (NAJAFI et al., 2015). All of these tests were used in our study, except for the tear osmolarity test, which is expensive, time-consuming and requires a lot of tears to be assessed, which is difficult in dry eye, and the microchip, which is more recent for analysing osmolarity, is not available in Brazil (NAJAFI et al., 2015).

In our study, we also used the OSDI (Ocular Surface Disease Index-Allergan) questionnaire (SCHIFFMAN et al., 2000), which is based on 12 questions about the presence and frequency of classic dry eye symptoms, the interference of symptoms with daily habits such as reading, watching television, driving and using a computer, and the worsening of symptoms in the presence of external factors such as strong wind, low humidity or exposure to air conditioning. This questionnaire generates a score, where dry eye is classified as normal, mild, moderate or severe dry eye. In the literature, the sensitivity and specificity of this questionnaire for diagnosing dry eye have been among the best when associated with the TRFL and the Schirmer test (ALVES et al., 2014), which were also used in our study.

The treatment of dry eye in these patients, as in other etiologies, has been difficult both because it is a multifactorial disease with a controversial diagnosis and because, in severe cases, the outcome has not been satisfactory (DRY EYE WORKSHOP, 2007c).

Conventional therapy includes various options such as artificial tears, occlusion of the lacrimal point, the use of therapeutic contact lenses and specific treatment of diseases of the ocular appendages. However, these therapies don't work for all patients. Surgical procedures such as the use of amniotic membranes and even corneal transplants have been carried out to restore damage to the ocular surface (ANITUA et al., 2015).

Artificial tears are by far the most widely used treatment. Among them are new formulations such as preservative-free, hypotonic, those containing lipids that prevent evaporation, substances with bioadhesive properties to increase water retention, and other formulas with protective substances against cellular stress caused by the hypertonicity of the tear (ARAGONA et al., 2013).

Studies have shown a relative improvement in patients with dry eye, especially when it comes to mild to moderate dry eye. A systematic review by Doughty et al. found that among all the types of artificial tears, such as hypromellose, polyacrylic acid and hyaluronic acid, there was an improvement in the signs of dry eye in approximately 25 per cent of cases, with no significant difference between the different groups of lubricants (DOUGHTY; GLAVIN, 2009). In our study, we found that of the 58 patients with moderate and severe dry eye, only 9 (15.52%) showed an improvement in symptoms with the previous use of lubricants, a difference probably attributable to the fact that our study only used diabetic patients, and the others used various dry eye etiologies.

Some studies have shown that the use of cyclosporine in dry eye reduces inflammation, but causes chronic eye irritation. Barreto et al. carried out a study comparing the use of cyclosporine with a lubricant (carboxymethylcellulose), and found no statistically significant difference between the two groups in terms of symptoms, corneal colour or LFTR; they only observed an improvement in the Schirmer test with cyclosporine (BARRETO et al., 2009). Only one of our patients had previously used cyclosporine, and we attribute this to the high cost of this medication. This patient had no improvement in symptoms or in the Schirmer test with this eye drop.

Corticosteroids have also had good results in some cases. Yang Chang et al. carried out a study with 30 patients who obtained improvement with the use of fluormethalone, but the side effects are important, such as the risk of developing cataracts and glaucoma (ANITUA et al., 2015; YANG; SUN; GU, 2006). Only one of the patients in this study had previously used this medication, and he didn't see any improvement in his dry eye and developed ocular hypertension after using it.

The big problem is that none of these treatments contain the properties of the human tear, especially without the bioactive molecules and growth factors (DOGRU; TSUBOTA, 2011). Then in 1975 Ralph et al reported a satisfactory effect of autologous serum in ocular surface diseases (RALPH; DOANE; DOHLMAN, 1975), reinforced in 1984 by Fox et al who used plasma in dry eye (FOX et al., 1984). Since then, it has been discovered that autologous serum maintains intracellular ATP and cell membrane integrity, which does not occur with artificial tears (POON et al., 2001).

Some authors have compared autologous serum with artificial tears and found an improvement in symptoms and clinical signs of dry eye with the former. Urzua et al, for example, carried out a double-blind randomised study comparing patients with artificial tears and serum, and assessed symptoms by OSDI, finding a 50% improvement for patients using autologous serum, in contrast to 22% in patients using artificial tears (URZUA et al., 2012). To date, there have been no randomised trials comparing platelet concentrate with artificial tears in dry eye, nor comparing the efficacy of autologous serum with platelet concentrate eye drops. In our study, what we observed was that all twelve patients showed total or partial improvement with CCP, and all reported that compared to the lubricants they had previously used, they had never seen such improvement in such a short space of time.

More recent studies have used plasma rich in growth factors or platelet-rich plasma, as they contribute to haemostasis, as well as containing numerous growth factors and cytokines that play a fundamental role in tissue regeneration. Their use was reported in 1990 with an adhesive function, similar to fibrin glue (GIBBLE; NESS, 1990). Once activated, platelets release an extensive number of proteins and growth factors such as PDGF, TGF-b, VEGF, IGF-I, HGF, PF-4, thrombospodin, angiopoetin, among others, initiating the healing process. As well as having many more growth factors than autologous serum, platelet concentrate has the advantage of having a greater number of platelets and no leucocytes, which trigger an inflammatory response (ANITUA et al., 2015).

In 2007, Alio et al. reported the use of platelet concentrate (PC) in a pilot study in 18 patients with symptomatic dry eye, with excellent improvement in symptoms and a reduction in corneal staining. In 2011, Lopez-Plandolit et al. described its use in 16 patients, also with good improvement in symptoms and some clinical signs. Both studies used patients with various causes of dry eye (ALIO et al., 2007a; LÓPEZ-PLANDOLIT et al., 2011). However, to date there have been no studies using this treatment in diabetic patients.

In our methodology, we used 12 diabetic patients, a similar number to the two existing studies on the use of CCP in dry eye from other causes. The statistics were based on patients rather than eyes, since dry eye disease is a pathology that generally occurs symmetrically in both eyes; and for some variables we used the average of the values between the two eyes, which provides less variability between measurements (RAY et al., 1985).

A sample size was calculated for the 221 diabetic patients, but the final sample size was by convenience. We didn't carry out a randomised study with a control group because the patients were already refractory to the usual treatments and had complications from the disease, so we intended to treat them. And this is a clinical trial study because we used a single group with the pathology, who underwent a treatment and were assessed before and after it.

Another controversial topic, which was used as an exclusion criterion, would be positive serological tests for blood-borne diseases. With the exception of HIV, where it is already known that the virus can reactivate when reinfused, the other diseases would not be a formal contraindication, since the donation would be autologous. However, because there is also the risk of contaminated material being handled by healthcare staff, it was decided not to treat these patients (GEERLING; MACLENNAN; HARTWIG, 2004).

Four patients out of the initial 25 were excluded due to positive serologies. This was a relatively high rate, given that, for example, a thesis carried out to evaluate positive serologies in a blood bank revealed that of more than 37,000 donors, 0.07% were HBSAg positive, 0.03% were HIV positive, and 0.13% were VDRL positive. In contrast to the findings of this study, we found that 8% (2/25) had HIV, 4% (1/25) syphilis, and 4% (1/25) HBSAg positive. However, the comparison is limited by the marked difference between the samples (FERREIRA, 2007).

Diabetes mellitus is not a contraindication for autologous donation as long as it is clinically compensated (MINISTÉRIO DA SAÚDE, 2001; BRASIL, 2013), but one limitation to treatment with CCP is impaired venous access; and 16% of patients (4/25) were unable to undergo treatment because we were unable to perform the puncture for donation. The same has been observed in the literature, and venous access difficulties occur more frequently in the elderly and diabetics (KONNER, 2000).

In their study, Alio et al. used the autologous donation technique to obtain platelet concentrates (ALIO et al., 2007a). Rezende et al, in their first report on the use of platelet concentrates in Brazil for neurotrophic ulcers after corneal transplantation, used the platelet apheresis technique (REZENDE et al., 2007).

It is known that there are more than 30 techniques for obtaining CCP, many of which are even commercialised. There is great variation in composition, protein content, amount of platelets, presence or absence of leucocytes, and also different indications for each one. This means that the results in terms of both efficacy and safety vary in the literature (ANITUA et al., 2015).

The ways in which platelet concentrate can be used, in addition to CCP, are in injectable form and as fibrin bioadhesives or fibrin membranes, with sealing properties, applied to ulcers or wounds on the ocular surface (ANITUA; TROYA; ORIVE, 2012).

With regard to the clinical results, 100 per cent of our patients showed an improvement in symptom complaints, such as dryness, burning, foreign body sensation, blurred vision and hyperemia; only one symptom, crusting and mucus, improved in the only two patients who had this complaint. This symptom of crusts and mucus could also be due to associated blepharitis, which can also contribute to dry eye.

The only two studies that reported the use of CCP in dry eye of various causes (but not specifically in diabetics) had similar findings: Alio et al observed that 89% of the 18 patients evolved with some total or partial improvement in symptoms; and Lopez-Plandolit et al found that 14 of the 16 patients evaluated (87.5%) (ALIO et al., 2007a; LÓPEZ-PLANDOLIT et al., 2011) obtained an improvement in the SDEQ 3 score (modified Dry Eye Questionnaire), 2011) obtained an improvement in the SDEQ 3 (modified Dry Eye Questionnaire) score, which is difficult to compare as the method used to assess it was different between the present study and the latter two, and these studies were carried out with patients with other dry eye aetiologies, mainly Sjogren's Syndrome and Stevens Jonhsons, whose dry eye mechanisms are different from those that occur in diabetic patients.

Following the DEWS severity table, once the symptoms have been assessed, the signs are then evaluated and the objective tests performed, which are the TRFL and the Schirmer test.

In the "conjunctival injection" item of the DEWS severity criteria, which generally means inflammation of the ocular surface, we assessed the degree of hyperaemia in our patients before and after treatment. Similar to the study by Alio et al (ALIO et al., 2007a), we found only 33.3% of patients who had this clinical sign before treatment, compatible with the first study which found 38.9% of patients who had the sign before treatment. Of these, 86% (6/7) improved after treatment, while in our study, all 4 patients who had the symptom before (100%) achieved clinical improvement.

It is very likely that surface inflammation has decreased in these patients, not only due to the dilution of pro-inflammatory factors on the ocular surface, but also due to inflammation inhibitors such as interleukin-1 receptor antagonists, metalloproteinase inhibitors and epithelial growth factor (ANITUA et al., 2004).

Conjunctival staining can be assessed with the three vital dyes, although if fluorescein is used, it would be ideal to use a specific yellow filter to improve contrast. The fluorescein stains the spaces where there is a loss of cellular integrity. Rose bengal can be used as well as lissamine green; both stain devitalised cells, mucus and filaments. Rose bengal colours the conjunctiva well, but is more toxic and irritating than lissamine green (QUEIROGA; DINIZ, 2010).

In our study, only 6 patients had some conjunctival colouration, using rose bengal 1% and fluorescein sodium 1%. All six had some improvement, following the DEWS severity gradation (DRY EYE WORKSHOP, 2007c). This topic was not evaluated in either of the two studies with CCP in dry eye.

Fluorescein staining of the cornea is an important parameter in the diagnosis and management of dry eye, as this disease can alter the ocular surface and cause damage to the corneal epithelium due to tear instability (GAYTON, 2009). The presence of keratitis was assessed in the study by Alio et al. and an improvement was found in 72 per cent of patients, all of whom had this sign before treatment. In our study, only two patients had this clinical sign, and both improved, as assessed by the DEWS severity criteria (DRY EYE WORKSHOP, 2007c).

Other signs in the cornea and tear film include *debris* in the tear, mucus and filaments, which are indications of tear instability, as well as alterations in the mucin and lipid layers. This criterion also takes into account the height of the tear meniscus, which is measured at the slit lamp and consists of the distance between the margin of the lower eyelid and the boundary between the ocular surface and the edge of the tear. Many authors consider it to be reduced when it is below 0.35mm (FRIDMAN, 2004), which was the parameter used in this study.

Among the 12 patients in this study, 83.33% had an improvement in the appearance of the tear film, in contrast to the 56% of cases in Alio et al. This difference may be attributed to the different etiologies of the cases in that study, where many patients with Sjogren's Syndrome and Stevens Johnson Syndrome were evaluated.

With regard to Meibomius gland dysfunction or eyelid alterations, it is known that patients with dry eye may have an eyelid or gland disease that can influence dry eye, either by causing increased evaporation or decreased tear secretion (BEHRENS et al., 2006). Only 3 had alterations before, and of these, (2/3) or 66.67% improved. One patient did not improve, as she had grade 4 of this sign, with trichiasis and eyelid scars. This criterion was not assessed in either of the other two studies using CCP in dry eye.

The Schirmer test is a test that generally evaluates the amount of tear secretion. In diabetics, this test has been shown to be altered (GOEBBELS, 2000; RAMOS-REMUS; SUAREZ-ALMAZOR; RUSSELL, 1994). Some authors do not consider it a good test in cases of evaporative dry eye (MCGINNIGLE; NAROO; EPERJESI, 2012), but other studies show that it is still one of the best tests, among those most commonly used in daily clinical practice, to detect dry eye, especially in diabetic patients (ALVES et al., 2014).

We preferred to assess the Schirmer test in two ways, both by following the gradation from 1 to 4 in the DEWS severity table (DRY EYE WORKSHOP, 2007c) and by analysing the average measurement in millimetres between the two eyes. The baseline test was carried out without anaesthetic. The Schirmer value, considering the gradation from 1 to 4, improved in 41.66% of patients, as the average Schirmer value before treatment was 6.75mm ± 3.66, and 8.96mm ± 4.56 after treatment ($P = 0.04$).

In this way, 66.67% (8/12) showed improvement in this test, 25% (3/12) had no change and 1 patient (8.33%) evolved with a lower test value after treatment. These results, when compared to the study by Lopez-Plandolit et al. (LÓPEZ-PLANDOLIT et al., 2011), are similar, as they found mean values of 4.67 ± 5.14 before and 6.91 ± 6.36 after.

The tear film break-up time (TRFL) or TBUT is related to tear stability, i.e. it is an appropriate test in diabetic patients because there is tear film instability, which has already been reported by some authors (JIN et al., 2003). It is even considered one of the best tests in terms of sensitivity and specificity for screening dry eye in diabetics (NAJAFI et al., 2015). We observed that 58.33 per cent had an improvement in TRFL, similar to the study by Alio et al. in which 50 per cent had an improvement (ALIO et al., 2007a).

Visual acuity was also analysed in all patients, using best corrected visual acuity, and it is known that any alterations to the ocular surface can lead to low visual acuity, including in cases of severe dry eye where lesions such as ulcers, leucomas and perforations can occur, with irreversible visual damage (MANAVIAT et al., 2008).

In our study, the gain in visual acuity lines occurred in 41.66% of patients. In the study by Alio et al. this gain in lines was 28 %, a disparity that can once again be explained by the diversity of dry eye etiologies, which are being compared here (ALIO et al., 2007a).

Of the 12 patients who also underwent the OSDI questionnaire before and after using CCP, all (100 per cent) saw an improvement in their scores after treatment. According to the mean score, before treatment the patients had severe dry eye and after treatment the mean score corresponded to mild dry eye. It was also observed that 50% progressed from some degree of dry eye to "normal" eye after treatment.

In Lopez-Plandolit's study, a different type of questionnaire was used, the SDEQ3, as mentioned above, making it difficult to compare the results, however these authors found an improvement of 87.5 per cent of symptoms after treatment, of which 43.75 per cent had an improvement assessed as "substantial", which in their study corresponds to a decrease of more than 50 per cent in the value of their score (LÓPEZ-PLANDOLIT et al., 2011).

In the study by Alio et al, there were 6 patients with severe dry eye (33.33%) and 12 (66.67%) with moderate dry eye before treatment, classified by the Madrid criteria, but they did not classify them after treatment. Lopez-Plandolit et al., although they described the value of their questionnaire scores before and after in their article, discuss the improvement in the score with CCP, but do not describe the final severity classification of these patients before and after. In our study, we initially had 12 patients, of whom 5 (41.67%) belonged to grade 2 of the DEWS severity table, 6 patients (50%) to grade or level 3 and 1 patient (8.33%) to grade 4.

The DEWS recommends that there should be at least one symptom and one clinical sign at each level in order to characterise it. We observed that 04 patients at level 2, for example, could also be classified as grade "3", since they had grade 3 symptoms, but all the objective signs and tests were grade 2 or lower. Using only the OSDI, we had one patient with moderate dry eye and 11 with severe dry eye.

After treatment, assessed by the DEWS criteria, 33.33% (4/12) had grade 1 dry eye, 4 (58.33%) had grade 2, and 1 patient (8.33%) had grade 3 dry eye. Evaluated by the OSDI, after treatment, 6 patients out of the 12 (50%) evaluated had a score classified as "normal", 4 of them (33.33%) for mild dry eye, 2 of them (16.67%) for moderate dry eye and one of them (8.33%) developed severe dry eye. It would be impossible to compare our results with the two studies above, as they both use different instruments and classification methods, and once again with patients with completely different aetiologies.

The classification, general approach, screening and follow-up of patients with dry eye are very subjective (DRY EYE WORKSHOP, 2007c), even when assessing clinical tests such as conjunctival staining, TFRL, conjunctival injection, corneal staining, presence and severity of meibomian dysfunction. In this study, two ophthalmologists assessed the patients in an attempt to reduce this bias.

The clinical importance of this study is that, as diabetic patients already have worsening of other associated comorbidities, dry eye can become more serious due to the vascular and neuropathic changes that occur, with the possibility of progressing to severe visual loss due to the complications of diabetes.

It is therefore clear how many patients with symptomatic dry eye have tried countless therapies without success. This is no different in diabetics, where a large proportion of patients are refractory to lubricants and other conventional treatments.

The efficacy of platelet-rich plasma in various areas of ophthalmology has been proven in the literature since the 1990s, with the aim of tissue regeneration and healing. And its use in dry eye has been described in two clinical trials, with very promising results. In addition to the numerous advantages of containing various growth factors, autologous PBC also has the advantage of avoiding the transmission of diseases and immunogenic reactions (OGINO et al., 2005).

There are no studies in the literature using CCP exclusively in the dry eye of diabetic patients, and we observed in this research that it could be a promising option to provide these patients with a better quality of life and reduce the morbidity of dry eye in this population, which is already so susceptible.

As for the complications reported in the literature with the use of CCP, they are extremely rare. Two cases of infection (LEITE et al., 2006), deposition of immunoglobulins in the cornea and keratic infiltrates have been reported in one case (MCDONNELL; SCHANZLIN; RAO, 1988). In our study, there were no complications. And there was good tolerance in all cases, so much so that when asked if they would repeat the treatment, the patients all said yes.

A limitation of the technique in our study was the fact that diabetic patients had more difficult peripheral venous access, which excluded 4 patients for this reason. Another limitation would be, for example, patients with serious comorbidities that contraindicate autologous donation, including anaemia (VANE; GANEM, 2006) (LÓPEZ-GARCÍA et al., 2007), but there is still the option of using serum rich in growth factors, obtained from the umbilical cord (VERSURA et al., 2015), i.e. heterologous.

Another limitation of this study was the fact that out of a sample of 221 patients, only 12 were able to undergo treatment, as the sample was lost due to the exclusions already discussed. However, this has been compatible with the literature, in which Alio et al studied a sample of 18 patients, and Lopez-Plandolit et al evaluated 16 patients.

The fact that it was an invasive treatment, where patients had to undergo venipuncture to donate blood, could indeed be a disadvantage, but what was observed in this study was that, given the severity of the symptoms of dry eye, which really interfered with the patients' daily activities and quality of life, none of them gave up on the treatment for this reason; on the contrary, knowing that the donation can be repeated every 4 months (VANE; GANEM, 2006), all twelve said they were willing to repeat it as many times as necessary (RIBEIRO et al, 2016).

In this study, the answer to the question was positive: we observed that treatment with CCP was effective in this group of patients, improving the symptoms and severity of dry eye in a large proportion of them.

CHAPTER 8

CONCLUSIONS

Epidemiologically, the patients with diabetic dry eye who came to our service had a mean age of 59.5 ± 11.58 years, more prevalent in females, with half of the patients being brown and having incomplete primary education and approximately 60 per cent earning up to one minimum wage.

Symptomatic dry eye occurred in approximately a quarter (58/221) of the diabetics who attended the ophthalmology service during the period of this study

After treatment with CCP, there was a significant improvement in the severity of dry eye in these patients, both when assessed by the OSDI, where half of the patients progressed to "normal", and by the DEWS, where approximately 83.33 per cent had a partial or total improvement in the gradation.

It can be concluded from these findings that the therapeutic response with CCP was indeed satisfactory in the dry eyes of diabetic patients who do not respond to conventional therapy. Randomised clinical trials are needed, however, so that standardised protocols for the production and use of this treatment can be created and these patients can be assessed over the long term.

REFERENCES

AKINCI, A.; CETINKAYA, E.; AYCAN, Z. Dry eye syndrome in diabetic children. European Journal of Ophthalmology, v. 17, n. 6, p. 873-878, dec. 2007.

ALIO, J. L. et al. Symptomatic dry eye treatment with autologous platelet-rich plasma. Ophthalmic Research, v. 39, n. 3, p. 124-129, 2007a.

ALIO, J. L. et al. Use of autologous platelet-rich plasma in the treatment of dormant corneal ulcers. Ophthalmology, v. 114, n. 7, p. 1286-1293.e1, jul. 2007b.

ALIO, J. L.; RODRIGUEZ, A. E.; WRÓBELDUDZINSKA, D. Eye platelet-rich plasma in the treatment of ocular surface disorders. Current Opinion in Ophthalmology, v. 26, n. 4, p. 325-332, jul. 2015.

ALVARADO VALERO, M. C. et al. Treatment of persistent epithelial defects using autologous serum application. Archivos De La Sociedad Espanola De Oftalmologia, v. 79, n. 11, p. 537-542, nov. 2004.

ALVES, M. et al. Comparison of diagnostic tests in distinct well-defined conditions related to dry eye disease. PloS One, v. 9, n. 5, p. e97921, 2014.

ALVES, M. DE C. et al. Tear film and ocular surface changes in diabetes mellitus. Arquivos Brasileiros de Oftalmologia, v. 71, n. 6, p. 96-103, dec. 2008.

AMERICAN ACADEMY OF OPHTHALMOLOGY. Dry Eye Syndrome Preferred Practice Pattern: Preferred Practice Patern. United States: AAO, 2013. Available at: <http://www.aao.

org/preferred-practice-pattern/dry-eye-syndrome- ppp--2013>.

AMERICAN DIABETES ASSOCIATION. (2) Classification and diagnosis of diabetes. Diabetes Care, v. 38 Suppl, p. S8-S16, jan. 2015.

ANDRESEN, J. L.; EHLERS, N. Chemotaxis of human keratocytes is increased by platelet-derived growth factor-BB, epidermal growth factor, transforming growth factor-alpha, acidic fibroblast growth factor, insulin-like growth factor-I, and transforming growth factor-beta. Current Eye Research, v. 17, n. 1, p. 79-87, jan. 1998.

ANITUA, E. et al. Autologous platelets as a source of proteins for healing and tissue regeneration. Thrombosis and Haemostasis, v. 91, n. 1, p. 4-15, jan. 2004.

ANITUA, E. et al. Autologous preparations rich in growth factors promote proliferation and induce VEGF and HGF production by human tendon cells in culture. Journal of Orthopaedic Research: Official Publication of the Orthopaedic Research Society, v. 23, n. 2, p. 281-286, mar. 2005.

ANITUA, E. et al. Plasma rich in growth factors (PRGF-Endoret) stimulates corneal wound healing and reduces haze formation after PRK surgery. Experimental Eye Research, v. 115, p. 153-161, Oct. 2013.

ANITUA, E. et al. Autologous serum and plasma rich in growth factors in ophthalmology: preclinical and clinical studies. Acta Ophthalmologica, 2 Apr. 2015.

ANITUA, E.; TROYA, M.; ORIVE, G. Plasma rich in growth factors promote gingival tissue regeneration by stimulating fibroblast proliferation and migration and by blocking transforming growth factor-01-mediated myodifferentiation. Journal of Periodontology, v. 83, n. 8, p. 1028-1037, Aug. 2012.

ARAGONA, P. et al. Effects of amino acids enriched tears substitutes on the cornea of patients with dysfunctional tear syndrome. Acta Ophthalmologica, v. 91, n. 6, p. e437 -|.|.|. sep. 2013.

AYRES, M. et al. BioEstat statistical applications in the bio-medical sciences, version 3.0. 2003. Belém: Sociedade Civil Mamirauá/MCT CNPq.[Links], [n.d.].

BARRETO, R. DE P. P. et al. Use of topical cyclosporine 0.05% in the treatment of dry eye in HIV-positive patients. Revista Brasileira de Oftalmologia, v. 68, n. 2, p. 83-89, Apr. 2009.

BEGLEY, C. G. et al. Use of the dry eye questionnaire to measure symptoms of ocular irritation in patients with aqueous tear deficient dry eye. Cornea, v. 21, n. 7, p. 664-670, oct. 2002.

BEHRENS, A. et al. Dysfunctional tear syndrome: a Delphi approach to treatment recommendations. Cornea, v. 25, n. 8, p. 900-907, sep. 2006.

BELFORT JR, R.; KARA-JOSE, N. Cornea: clinical and surgical. São Paulo: Roca, 1997.

BINDER, A. et al. Sjogren's syndrome: association with type-1 diabetes mellitus. British Journal of Rheumatology, v. 28, n. 6, p. 518-520, dec. 1989.

BLOMQUIST, P. H. Ocular complications of systemic medications. The American Journal of the Medical Sciences, v. 342, n. 1, p. 62-69, Jul. 2011.

BOSCO, A. et al. Diabetic retinopathy. Arquivos Brasileiros de Endocrinologia & Metabologia, v. 49, n. 2, p. 217-227, Apr. 2005.

BRAZIL. Ministry of Health. Ordinance 2712, of 12 November 2013. Federal Official Gazette. n 221. Brasília, 13 November 2013.

BREWITT, H.; SISTANI, F. Dry eye disease: the scale of the problem. Survey of Ophthalmology, v. 45 Suppl 2, p. S199-202, mar. 2001.

BRON, A. J.; TIFFANY, J. M. The contribution of meibomian disease to dry eye. The Ocular Surface, v. 2, n. 2, p. 149-165, Apr. 2004.

CAFFERY, B. E. et al. CANDEES. The Canadian Dry Eye Epidemiology Study. Advances in Experimental Medicine and Biology, v. 438, p. 805-806, 1998.

CAVALLI-SFORZA, L. L. Genes, peoples and languages. São Paulo: Companhia das Letras, 2003.

CHO, P. et al. Tear break-up time: clinical procedures and their effects. Ophthalmic & Physiological Optics: The Journal of the British College of Ophthalmic Opticians (Optometrists), v. 18, n. 4, p. 319-324, jul. 1998.

DEL CASTILLO, J. M. B. et al. Treatment of recurrent corneal erosions using autologous serum. Cornea, v. 21, n. 8, p. 781-783, nov. 2002.

DE PAIVA, C. S. et al. Corticosteroid and doxycycline suppress MMP-9 and inflammatory cytokine expression, MAPK activation in the corneal epithelium in experimental dry eye. Experimental Eye Research, v. 83, n. 3, p. 526-535, sep. 2006.

DOGRU, M.; TSUBOTA, K. Pharmacotherapy of dry eye. Expert Opinion on Pharmacotherapy, v. 12, n. 3, p. 325-334, feb. 2011.

DOUGHTY, M. J.; GLAVIN, S. Efficacy of different dry eye treatments with artificial tears or ocular lubricants: a systematic review. Ophthalmic & Physiological Optics: The Journal of the British College of Ophthalmic Opticians (Optometrists), v. 29, n. 6, p. 573-583, nov. 2009.

DRY EYE WORKSHOP. The definition and classification of dry eye disease: report of the Definition and Classification Subcommittee of the International Dry Eye WorkShop. The Ocular Surface, v. 5, n. 2, p. 75-92, abr. 2007a.

DRY EYE WORKSHOP. The epidemiology of dry eye disease: report of the Epidemiology Subcommittee of the International Dry Eye WorkShop. The Ocular Surface, v. 5, n. 2, p. 93-107, Apr. 2007b.

DRY EYE WORKSHOP. Methodologies to diagnose and monitor dry eye disease: report of the Diagnostic Methodology Subcommittee of the International Dry Eye WorkShop. The Ocular Surface, v. 5, n. 2, p. 108-152, Apr. 2007c.

FARRIS, R. L. Tear osmolarity--a new gold standard? Advances in Experimental Medicine and Biology, v. 350, p. 495-503, 1994.

FERREIRA, O. Estudo de doadores de sangue com serologia reagente para hepatites B e C,

HIV e sífilis no Hemocentro de Ribeirão Preto. text-[s.l.] Universidade de São Paulo, 27 Apr. 2007.

FERRIS, F. Early photocoagulation in patients with either type I or type II diabetes. Transactions of the American Ophthalmological Society, v. 94, p. 505-537, 1996.

FONSECA, E. C.; ARRUDA, G. V.; ROCHA, E. M. Dry eye: etiopathogenesis and treatment. Arq Bras Oftalmol, p. 197-203, 2010.

FOX, R. I. et al. Beneficial effect of artificial tears made with autologous serum in patients with keratoconjunctivitis sicca. Arthritis and Rheumatism, v. 27, n. 4, p. 459-461, Apr. 1984.

FREIRE, V. et al. In vitro effects of three blood derivatives on human corneal epithelial cells. Investigative Ophthalmology & Visual Science, v. 53, n. 9, p. 5571-5578, 2012.

FRIDMAN, D. Association between corneal hypoaesthesia, dry eye and other factors in patients with type 2 diabetes mellitus. Master's Thesis-Porto Alegre: Federal University of Rio Grande do Sul, 2004.

FUJISHIMA, H. et al. Allergic conjunctivitis and dry eye. The British Journal of Ophthalmology, v. 80, n. 11, p. 994-997, nov. 1996.

FUNG, M. K. et al. Technical manual. Bethesda, Md.: American Association of Blood Banks, 2014.

GALOR, A. et al. Prevalence and risk factors of dry eye syndrome in a United States veterans affairs population. American Journal of Ophthalmology, v. 152, n. 3, p. 377-384.e2, sep. 2011.

GAYTON, J. L. Etiology, prevalence, and treatment of dry eye disease. Clinical Ophthalmology (Auckland, N.Z.), v. 3, p. 405-412, 2009.

GEERLING, G.; MACLENNAN, S.; HARTWIG, D. Autologous serum eye drops for ocular surface disorders. The British Journal of Ophthalmology, v. 88, n. 11, p. 1467-1474, nov. 2004.

GIBBLE, J. W.; NESS, P. M. Fibrin glue: the perfect operative sealant? Transfusion, v. 30, n. 8, p. 741-747, Oct. 1990.

GOEBBELS, M. Tear secretion and tear film function in insulin dependent diabetics. The British Journal of Ophthalmology, v. 84, n. 1, p. 19-21, jan. 2000.

GOMES, B. et al. Signs and symptoms of ocular surface disease in patients on topical intraocular pressure-lowering therapy. Arquivos Brasileiros de Oftalmologia, v. 76, n. 5, p. 282-287, Oct. 2013.

GOTO, E. et al. Treatment of superior limbic keratoconjunctivitis by application of autologous serum. Cornea, v. 20, n. 8, p. 807-810, nov. 2001.

GUO, B. et al. Prevalence of dry eye disease in Mongolians at high altitude in China: the Henan eye study. Ophthalmic Epidemiology, v. 17, n. 4, p. 234-241, Aug. 2010.

HESS, K. The vulnerable blood. Coagulation and clot structure in diabetes mellitus.

Hamostaseologie, p. 25-33, 2015.

HOLZER, M. P. et al. Combination of transepithelial phototherapeutic keratectomy and autologous serum eyedrops for treatment of recurrent corneal erosions. Journal of Cataract and Refractive Surgery, v. 31, n. 8, p. 1603-1606, Aug. 2005.

HOM, M.; DE LAND, P. Self-reported dry eyes and diabetic history. Optometry (St. Louis, Mo.), v. 77, n. 11, p. 554-558, nov. 2006.

SYRIAN LEBANESE HOSPITAL. Guide to Haemotherapy Procedures. São Paulo: Syrian Lebanese Hospital, 2010.

HYON, J. Y.; LEE, Y. J.; YUN, P.-Y. Management of ocular surface inflammation in Sjogren's syndrome. Cornea, v. 26, n. 9 Suppl 1, p. S13-15, Oct. 2007.

IBGE. 2010 Demographic Census. Available at: <http://www.censo2010.ibge.gov.br/>. Accessed on: 18 August 2015.

JAVALOY, J. et al. Effect of platelet-rich plasma in nerve regeneration after LASIK. Journal of Refractive Surgery (Thorofare, N.J.: 1995), v. 29, n. 3, p. 213-219, Mar. 2013.

JEGANATHAN, V. S. E.; WANG, J. J.; WONG, T. Y. Ocular associations of diabetes other than diabetic retinopathy. Diabetes Care, v. 31, n. 9, p. 1905-1912, sep. 2008.

JIN, J. et al. [Tear film function in non-insulin dependent diabetics] [Zhonghua Yan Ke Za Zhi] Chinese Journal of Ophthalmology, v. 39, n. 1, p. 10-13, Jan. 2003.

JONNES, N. Substantially neutral aqueous lubricant. United States, U.S. Patent 4,461,712, 1984, Jul 24.

KAISERMAN, I. et al. Dry eye in diabetic patients. American Journal of Ophthalmology, v. 139, n. 3, p. 498-503, mar. 2005.

KHAKSAR, E. et al. The effect of sub-conjunctival platelet-rich plasma in combination with topical acetylcysteine on corneal alkali burn ulcer in rabbits.
Comparative Clinical Pathology, v. 22, n. 1, p. 107-112, 13 Dec. 2011.

KIM, K. M.; SHIN, Y.-T.; KIM, H. K. Effect of autologous platelet-rich plasma on persistent corneal epithelial defect after infectious keratitis. Japanese Journal of Ophthalmology, v. 56, n. 6, p. 544-550, nov. 2012.

KLENKLER, B.; SHEARDOWN, H.; JONES, L. Growth factors in the tear film: role in tissue maintenance, wound healing, and ocular pathology. The Ocular Surface, v. 5, n. 3, p. 228-239, jul. 2007.

KOFFLER, B. H. Autologous serum therapy of the ocular surface with novel delivery by platelet concentrate gel. The Ocular Surface, v. 4, n. 4, p. 188-195, oct. 2006.

KOJIMA, T. et al. The effect of autologous serum eyedrops in the treatment of severe dry eye disease: a prospective randomised case-control study. American Journal of Ophthalmology, v. 139, n. 2, p. 242-246, feb. 2005.

KONNER, K. Primary vascular access in diabetic patients: an audit. Nephrology Dialysis Transplantation, v. 15, n. 9, p. 1317-1325, 9 Jan. 2000.

LAWRENCE, M. S. et al. The D1 receptor antagonist, SCH 23390, induces signs of parkinsonism in African green monkeys. Life Sciences, v. 49, n. 25, p. PL229-234, 1991.

LEE, A. J. et al. Prevalence and risk factors associated with dry eye symptoms: a population based study in Indonesia. The British Journal of Ophthalmology, v. 86, n. 12, p. 1347-1351, dec. 2002.

LEE, G. A.; CHEN, S. X. Autologous serum in the management of recalcitrant dry eye syndrome. Clinical & Experimental Ophthalmology, v. 36, n. 2, p. 119-122, mar. 2008.

LEITE, S. C. et al. Risk factors and characteristics of ocular complications, and efficacy of autologous serum tears after haematopoietic progenitor cell transplantation. Bone Marrow Transplantation, v. 38, n. 3, p. 223-227, aug. 2006.

LEMP, M. A. Report of the National Eye Institute/Industry workshop on Clinical Trials in Dry Eyes. The CLAO journal: official publication of the Contact Lens Association of Ophthalmologists, Inc, v. 21, n. 4, p. 221-232, Oct. 1995.

LIU, L. et al. An optimised protocol for the production of autologous serum eyedrops. Graefe's Archive for Clinical and Experimental Ophthalmology, v. 243, n. 7, p. 706-714, jul. 2005.

LIU, L. et al. Corneal epitheliotrophic capacity of three different blood-derived preparations. Investigative Ophthalmology & Visual Science, v. 47, n. 6, p. 24382444, jun. 2006.

LÓPEZ-GARCÍA, J. S. et al. Use of autologous serum in ophthalmic practice. Archivos De La Sociedad Espanola De Oftalmologia, v. 82, n. 1, p. 9-20, jan. 2007.

LÓPEZ-GARCÍA, J. S. et al. Autologous serum eyedrops in the treatment of aniridic keratopathy. Ophthalmology, v. 115, n. 2, p. 262-267, feb. 2008.

LÓPEZ-GARCÍA, J. S. et al. Autologous serum eye drops diluted with sodium hyaluronate: clinical and experimental comparative study. Acta Ophthalmologica, v. 92, n. 1, p. e22-29, feb. 2014.

LÓPEZ-PLANDOLIT, S. et al. Efficacy of plasma rich in growth factors for the treatment of dry eye. Cornea, p. 1312-7, 2011.

MANAVIAT, M. R. et al. Prevalence of dry eye syndrome and diabetic retinopathy in type 2 diabetic patients. BMC Ophthalmology, v. 8, p. 10, 2 Jun. 2008.

MARASCHIN, J. DE F. et al. Diabetes mellitus classification. Arquivos Brasileiros de Cardiologia, v. 95, n. 2, p. 40-46, Aug. 2010.

MARQUEZ DE ARACENA DEL CID, R.; MONTERO DE ESPINOSA ESCORIAZA, I. Subconjunctival application of regenerative factor-rich plasma for the treatment of ocular alkali burns. European Journal of Ophthalmology, v. 19, n. 6, p. 909-915, dec. 2009.

MATSUMOTO, Y. et al. Autologous serum application in the treatment of neurotrophic keratopathy. Ophthalmology, v. 111, n. 6, p. 1115-1120, jun. 2004.

MATSUO, H. et al. Topical application of autologous serum for the treatment of late- onset aqueous oozing or point-leak through filtering bleb. Eye, v. 19, n. 1, p. 23-28, jan. 2005.

MATSUURA, N. et al. Predominance of infiltrating IL-4-producing T cells in conjunctiva of patients with allergic conjunctival disease. Current Eye Research, v. 29, n. 4-5, p. 235-243, nov. 2004.

MAVRAKANAS, N. A.; KIEL, R.; DOSSO, A. A. Autologous serum application in the treatment of Mooren's ulcer. Klinische Monatsblätter Fur Augenheilkunde, v. 224, n. 4, p. 300-302, Apr. 2007.

MCDONNELL, P. J.; SCHANZLIN, D. J.; RAO, N. A. Immunoglobulin deposition in the cornea after application of autologous serum. Archives of Ophthalmology, v. 106, n. 10, p. 1423-1425, Oct. 1988.

MCGINNIGLE, S.; NAROO, S. A.; EPERJESI, F. Evaluation of dry eye. Survey of Ophthalmology, v. 57, n. 4, p. 293-316, Aug. 2012.

MCMONNIES, C. W.; HO, A. Conjunctival hyperaemia in non-contact lens wearers. Acta Ophthalmologica, v. 69, n. 6, p. 799-801, 27 May 2009.

MESSMER, E. M. The Pathophysiology, Diagnosis, and Treatment of Dry Eye Disease. Deutsches Arzteblatt International, v. 112, n. 5, p. 71-82, Jan. 2015.

MINISTRY OF HEALTH. National Coordination of Sexually Transmitted Diseases and AIDS. Clinical Screening of Blood Donors. Brasília: Ministry of Health, 2001.

MINISTRY OF HEALTH. Health Care Secretariat. Primary Care Department. Diabetes Mellitus. Brasília: Ministry of Health, 2006.

MISRA, S. L. et al. Peripheral Neuropathy and Tear Film Dysfunction in Type 1 Diabetes Mellitus. Journal of Diabetes Research, v. 2014, 2014.

MIXON, B. et al. Autologous serum eye drops for severe dry eye syndrome in a patient with chronic graft-versus-host disease: a case report. International Journal of Pharmaceutical Compounding, v. 18, n. 5, p. 370-377, Oct. 2014.

MÓDULO, C. M. et al. Influence of insulin treatment on the lacrimal gland and ocular surface of diabetic rats. Endocrine, v. 36, n. 1, p. 161-168, Aug. 2009.

MOSS, S. E.; KLEIN, R.; KLEIN, B. E. Prevalence of and risk factors for dry eye syndrome. Archives of Ophthalmology, v. 118, n. 9, p. 1264-1268, sep. 2000.

MOSS, S. E.; KLEIN, R.; KLEIN, B. E. K. Incidence of dry eye in an older population. Archives of Ophthalmology, v. 122, n. 3, p. 369-373, mar. 2004.

MOSS, S. E.; KLEIN, R.; KLEIN, B. E. K. Long-term incidence of dry eye in an older population. Optometry and Vision Science: Official Publication of the American Academy of Optometry, v. 85, n. 8, p. 668-674, Aug. 2008.

MUNOZ B et al. Causes of blindness and visual impairment in a population of older americans: The salisbury eye evaluation study. Archives of Ophthalmology, v. 118, n. 6, p. 819-825, 1 Jun. 2000.

MURUBE, J. Classification of Dry Eye. In: SIMPÓSIO OLHO SECO. São Paulo: Medicopea, 2000

MURUBE, J. et al. The Madrid triple classification of dry eye. Archivos De La Sociedad Espanola De Oftalmologia, v. 78, n. 11, p. 587-593; 595-601, nov. 2003.

MURUBE, J. Tear osmolarity. The Ocular Surface, v. 4, n. 2, p. 62-73, Apr. 2006.

MY, A. Restoration of human lacrimal function following platelet-rich plasma injection. Cornea, p. 18-21, 2014.

NAJAFI, L. et al. Dry eye and its correlation to diabetes microvascular complications in people with type 2 diabetes mellitus. Journal of Diabetes and Its Complications, v. 27, n. 5, p. 459-462, Oct. 2013.

NAJAFI, L. et al. Dry eye disease in type 2 diabetes mellitus; comparison of the tear osmolarity test with other common diagnostic tests: a diagnostic accuracy study using STARD standard. Journal of Diabetes and Metabolic Disorders, v. 14, p. 39, 2015.

NARANJO, R. Dry eye: concept and treatment. In: SIMPÓSIO OLHO SECO. São Paulo: Medicopea, 2000

NEGI, A.; VERNON, S. A. An overview of the eye in diabetes. Journal of the Royal Society of Medicine, v. 96, n. 6, p. 266-272, jun. 2003.

NEPP, J. et al. Is there a correlation between the severity of diabetic retinopathy and keratoconjunctivitis sicca? Cornea, v. 19, n. 4, p. 487-491, jul. 2000.

NICHOLS, J. J. et al. The performance of the contact lens dry eye questionnaire as a screening survey for contact lens-related dry eye. Cornea, v. 21, n. 5, p. 469-475, jul. 2002.

NICHOLS, K. K.; NICHOLS, J. J.; MITCHELL, G. L. The reliability and validity of McMonnies Dry Eye Index. Cornea, v. 23, n. 4, p. 365-371, May 2004.

NOBLE, B. A. et al. Comparison of autologous serum eye drops with conventional therapy in a randomised controlled crossover trial for ocular surface disease. The British Journal of Ophthalmology, v. 88, n. 5, p. 647-652, May 2004.

NODA-TSURUYA, T. et al. Autologous serum eye drops for dry eyes after LASIK. Journal of Refractive Surgery (Thorofare, N.J.: 1995), v. 22, n. 1, p. 61-66, feb. 2006.

OGINO, Y. et al. The effect of platelet-rich plasma on the cellular response of rat bone marrow cells in vitro. Oral Surgery, Oral Medicine, Oral Pathology, Oral Radiology, and Endodontics, v. 100, n. 3, p. 302-307, sep. 2005.

PANDA, A. et al. Topical autologous platelet-rich plasma eyedrops for acute corneal chemical injury. Cornea, v. 31, n. 9, p. 989-993, sep. 2012.

PAN, Q. et al. Autologous serum eye drops for dry eye. The Cochrane Database of Systematic Reviews, v. 8, p. CD009327, 2013.

PEREIRA, G. A. B.; ARCHER, R. L. B.; RUIZ, C. A. C. Evaluation of the knowledge that patients with diabetes mellitus demonstrate about ocular changes due to this illness. Arquivos Brasileiros de Oftalmologia, v. 72, n. 4, p. 481-485, Aug. 2009.

PEREIRA GOMES, J. A.; LIMA, A. L.; ADAN, C. B. Normal Assessment of the Ocular Surface. In: ALVES, M. R.; LIMA, A. L. H.; DANTAS, M. C. N. (Eds.) . CBO Manual - External eye diseases and cornea. São Paulo: Cultura Médica, 1999.

PEZZOTTA, S. et al. Autologous platelet lysate for treatment of refractory ocular GVHD. Bone Marrow Transplantation, v. 47, n. 12, p. 1558-1563, dec. 2012.

PHAN, T. M. et al. Topical fibronectin in an alkali burn model of corneal ulceration in rabbits. Archives of Ophthalmology, v. 109, n. 3, p. 414-419, mar. 1991.

PHARMAKAKIS, N. M. et al. Corneal complications following abuse of topical anaesthetics. European Journal of Ophthalmology, v. 12, n. 5, p. 373-378, oct. 2002.

PISELLA, P. J.; POULIQUEN, P.; BAUDOUIN, C. Prevalence of ocular symptoms and signs with preserved and preservative free glaucoma medication. The British Journal of Ophthalmology, v. 86, n. 4, p. 418-423, Apr. 2002.

POON, A. C. et al. Autologous serum eyedrops for dry eyes and epithelial defects: clinical and in vitro toxicity studies. The British Journal of Ophthalmology, v. 85, n. 10, p. 1188-1197, Oct. 2001.

PORTAL BRASIL. Diabetes. News. Available at: <http://www.brasil.gov.br/saude/2012/04/diabetes>. Accessed on: 19 July 2015.

QUEIROGA, I. B. W. D.; DINIZ, M. D. F. F. M. Rose Bengal Ocular Surface Staining and the Diagnosis of Dry Eye. Revista Brasileira de Ciências da Saúde, v. 12, n. 1, p. 95-102, 31 Mar. 2010.

QUINTO, G. G.; CAMPOS, M.; BEHRENS, A. Autologous serum for ocular surface diseases: [review]. Arquivos Brasileiros de Oftalmologia, p. 47-54, 2008.

RAHMAN, A. et al. Diagnostic value of tear films tests in type 2 diabetes. JPMA. The Journal of the Pakistan Medical Association, v. 57, n. 12, p. 577-581, dec. 2007.

RALPH, R. A.; DOANE, M. G.; DOHLMAN, C. H. Clinical experience with a mobile ocular perfusion pump. Archives of Ophthalmology, v. 93, n. 10, p. 10391043, oct. 1975.

RAMOS-REMUS, C.; SUAREZ-ALMAZOR, M.; RUSSELL, A. S. Low tear production in patients with diabetes mellitus is not due to Sjõgren's syndrome.
Clinical and Experimental Rheumatology, v. 12, n. 4, p. 375-380, aug. 1994.

RAY, W. A. et al. Statistical analysis for experimental models of ocular disease: continuous response measures. Current Eye Research, v. 4, n. 5, p. 585-597, May 1985.

RAZOUK, F. H.; REICHE, E. M. V. Characterisation, production and indication of the principal blood components. Revista Brasileira de Hematologia e Hemoterapia, v. 26, n. 2, p. 126-134, jan. 2004.

REIDY, J. J.; PAULUS, M. P.; GONA, S. Recurrent erosions of the cornea: epidemiology and treatment. Cornea, v. 19, n. 6, p. 767-771, nov. 2000.

REZENDE, M. S. V. M. et al. Use of platelet concentrate in ocular surface disease. Brazilian Journal of Ophthalmology, p. 257-261, 2007.

RIBEIRO, M. V. M. R. et al. Platelet-rich plasma in diabetic dry eye disease. Brazilian Journal of Ophthalmology, v. 75, p. 308-313 2016.

RIORDAN-EVA, P.; WHITCHER, J. Vaughan & Asbury's general ophthalmology. [s.l.] Wiley Online Library, 2008.

SCHAUMBERG, D. A. et al. Prevalence of dry eye disease among US men: estimates from the Physicians' Health Studies. Archives of Ophthalmology, v. 127, n. 6, p. 763-768, jun. 2009.

SCHEIN, O. D. et al. Prevalence of dry eye among the elderly. American Journal of Ophthalmology, v. 124, n. 6, p. 723-728, dec. 1997.

SCHEIN, O. D. et al. Dry eye and dry mouth in the elderly: a population-based assessment. Archives of Internal Medicine, v. 159, n. 12, p. 1359-1363, 28 Jun. 1999.

SCHIFFMAN, R. M. et al. Reliability and validity of the Ocular Surface Disease Index. Archives of Ophthalmology, v. 118, n. 5, p. 615-621, May 2000.

SEIFART, U.; STREMPEL, I. [The dry eye and diabetes mellitus]. Der Ophthalmologe: Zeitschrift Der Deutschen Ophthalmologischen Gesellschaft, v. 91, n. 2, p. 235-239, Apr. 1994.

SENDECKA, M.; BARYLUK, A.; POLZ-DACEWICZ, M. [Prevalence and risk factors of dry eye syndrome]. Przegl^id Epidemiologiczny, v. 58, n. 1, p. 227-233, 2004.

SERRARBASSA, P. D.; DIAS, A. F. G.; VIEIRA, M. F. New concepts on diabetic retinopathy: neural versus vascular damage. Arquivos Brasileiros de Oftalmologia, v. 71, n. 3, p. 459-463, jun. 2008.

SHARMA, N. et al. Evaluation of umbilical cord serum therapy in acute ocular chemical burns. Investigative Ophthalmology & Visual Science, v. 52, n. 2, p. 1087-1092, feb. 2011.

SHIMMURA, S. et al. Albumin as a tear supplement in the treatment of severe dry eye. The British Journal of Ophthalmology, v. 87, n. 10, p. 1279-1283, Oct. 2003.

SHIMMURA, S.; SHIMAZAKI, J.; TSUBOTA, K. Results of a population-based questionnaire on the symptoms and lifestyles associated with dry eye. Cornea, v. 18, n. 4, p. 408-411, jul. 1999.

SHRESTHA, R. K. Ocular manifestations in diabetes, a hospital based prospective study. Nepal Medical College journal: NMCJ, v. 13, n. 4, p. 254-256, dec. 2011.

SMITH, J. The epidemiology of dry eye disease. Acta Ophthalmologica Scandinavica, v. 85, 2007.

STERN, M. E. et al. The pathology of dry eye: the interaction between the ocular surface and lacrimal glands. Cornea, v. 17, n. 6, p. 584-589, nov. 1998.

SULLIVAN, D. A. et al. Do sex steroids exert sex-specific and/or opposite effects on gene expression in lacrimal and meibomian glands? Molecular Vision, v. 15, p. 1553-1572, 2009.

TANANUVAT, N. et al. Controlled study of the use of autologous serum in dry eye patients. Cornea, v. 20, n. 8, p. 802-806, nov. 2001.

TEI, M. et al. Vitamin A deficiency alters the expression of mucin genes by the rat ocular surface epithelium. Investigative Ophthalmology & Visual Science, v. 41, n. 1, p. 82-88, jan. 2000.

TIAN, Y.-J. et al. [Epidemiological study of dry eye in populations equal or over 20 years old in Jiangning District of Shanghai]. [Zhonghua Yan Ke Za Zhi] Chinese Journal of Ophthalmology, v. 45, n. 6, p. 486-491, jun. 2009.

TOKER, E.; ASFUROGLU, E. Corneal and conjunctival sensitivity in patients with dry eye: the effect of topical cyclosporine therapy. Cornea, v. 29, n. 2, p. 133-140, feb. 2010.

TOMLINSON, A. et al. Tear film osmolarity: determination of a referent for dry eye diagnosis. Investigative Ophthalmology & Visual Science, v. 47, n. 10, p. 43094315, oct. 2006.

TSUBOTA, K. et al. Surgical reconstruction of the ocular surface in advanced ocular cicatricial pemphigoid and Stevens-Johnson syndrome. American Journal of Ophthalmology, v. 122, n. 1, p. 38-52, jul. 1996.

TSUBOTA, K. et al. Treatment of dry eye by autologous serum application in Sjõgren's syndrome. The British Journal of Ophthalmology, v. 83, n. 4, p. 390- 395, Apr. 1999a.

TSUBOTA, K. et al. Treatment of persistent corneal epithelial defect by autologous serum application. Ophthalmology, v. 106, n. 10, p. 1984-1989, oct. 1999b.

UNTERLAUFT, J. D. et al. Albumin eye drops for treatment of ocular surface diseases. Der Ophthalmologe: Zeitschrift Der Deutschen Ophthalmologischen Gesellschaft, v. 106, n. 10, p. 932-937, Oct. 2009.

URZUA, C. A. et al. Randomised double-blind clinical trial of autologous serum versus artificial tears in dry eye syndrome. Current Eye Research, v. 37, n. 8, p. 684-688, Aug. 2012.

VAN BIJSTERVELD, O. P. Diagnostic tests in the Sicca syndrome. Archives of Ophthalmology, v. 82, n. 1, p. 10-14, jul. 1969.

VANE, L. A.; GANEM, E. M. Homologous versus Autologous Donation and Haemoglobin Substitutes. In: CAVALCANTI, I. L.; CANTINHO, F. A. DE F.; ASSAD, A. (Eds.). Perioperative Medicine. Rio de Janeiro: SAERJ, 2006. p. 291-306.

VERSURA, P. et al. Targeting growth factor supply in keratopathy treatment: comparison between maternal peripheral blood and cord blood as sources for the preparation of topical eye drops. Blood Transfusion, p. 1-7, 9 Jul. 2015.

VERSURA, P.; PROFAZIO, V.; CAMPOS, E. C. Performance of Tear Osmolarity Compared to Previous Diagnostic Tests for Dry Eye Diseases. Current Eye Research, v. 35, n. 7, p. 553-564, 1 Jul. 2010.

VICK, V. L. et al. Use of autologous platelet concentrate in blepharoplasty surgery. Ophthalmic

Plastic and Reconstructive Surgery, v. 22, n. 2, p. 102-104, Apr. 2006.

WAKAMATSU, T. H.; DOGRU, M.; TSUBOTA, K. Tearful relations: oxidative stress, inflammation and eye diseases: [review]. Arquivos Brasileiros de Oftalmologia, p. 72-79, 2008.

WANG, Y. et al. Ocular surface and tear functions after topical cyclosporine treatment in dry eye patients with chronic graft-versus-host disease. Bone Marrow Transplantation, v. 41, n. 3, p. 293-302, feb. 2008.

WOOST, P. G. et al. Growth factors and corneal endothelial cells: II. Characterisation of epidermal growth factor receptor from bovine corneal endothelial cells. Cornea, v. 11, n. 1, p. 11-19, jan. 1992.

WORLD MEDICAL ASSOCIATION. World Medical Association Declaration of Helsinki: ethical principles for medical research involving human subjects. JAMA, v. 310, n. 20, p. 2191-2194, 27 Nov. 2013.

XU, K. P. et al. Tear function index. A new measure of dry eye. Archives of Ophthalmology, v. 113, n. 1, p. 84-88, jan. 1995.

YAMADA, N. et al. Role of the C domain of IGFs in synergistic promotion, with a substance P-derived peptide, of rabbit corneal epithelial wound healing. Investigative Ophthalmology & Visual Science, v. 45, n. 4, p. 1125-1131, Apr. 2004.

YANG, C.; SUN, W.; GU, Y. A clinical study of the efficacy of topical corticosteroids on dry eye. Journal of Zhejiang University. Science. B, v. 7, n. 8, p. 675-678, Aug. 2006.

YANG, H. Y. et al. Lacrimal punctal occlusion for the treatment of superior limbic keratoconjunctivitis. American Journal of Ophthalmology, v. 124, n. 1, p. 80-87, Jul. 1997.

YAO, K. et al. Efficacy of 1% carboxymethylcellulose sodium for treating dry eye after phacoemulsification: results from a multicenter, open-label, randomized, controlled study. BMC ophthalmology, v. 15, p. 28, 2015.

YOON, K.-C. et al. Comparison of autologous serum and umbilical cord serum eye drops for dry eye syndrome. American Journal of Ophthalmology, v. 144, n. 1, p. 86-92, jul. 2007.

YOUNG, A. L. et al. The use of autologous serum tears in persistent corneal epithelial defects. Eye, v. 18, n. 6, p. 609-614, jun. 2004.

APPENDIX A - Questionnaire

Diabetic patients - use of platelet concentrate in dry eye.

GLYCEMIA JEJUM
GLYCATED HGB
PROTEIN

Questionnaire

Name:

Record and location: age

Sex: Colour:

Phone:

1.	Severe heart disease or recent revascularisation:	S( )	N( )
2.	Contact lens wearer	S( )	N( )
3.	Corneal disease (such as oedema)	S( )	N( )
4.	STROKE	S()	N( )
5.	Dementia or disabling neurological/psychiatric illness	S()	N( )
6.	Use of medication. Which	S()	N( )
7.	Have you ever had a laser for diabetic retinopathy?	S()	N( )
8.	Had eye surgery	S()	N( )
9.	Use any eye drops	S()	N( )
10.	Smoke	S()	N( )
11.	Rheumatic disease	S()	N( )
12.	Thyroid disease	S()	N( )
13.	Inflammatory bowel disease	S()	N( )
14.	Bronchitis / asthma / allergies	S()	N( )
15.	Mouth or other dry mucosa	S()	N( )
16.	Eye diseases	S()	N( )

SYMPTOMS OF DRY EYE / **DEWS**

a)	Dry eyes	never	a few times	frequent	constant
b)	Burning/sand sensation	never	a few times	frequent	constant
c)	Burning	never	a few times	frequent	constant
d)	Redness	never	a few times	frequent	constant
e)	Crusty eyelashes	never	a few times	frequent	constant
f)	Eyes stuck together in the morning	never	a few times	frequent	constant
g)	Visual symptoms	never	a few times	frequent	constant

TO THE EXAM / DEWS

CONJUNCTIVAL INJECTION **ABSENT ()** MIGHT () MODERATE () SERIOUS ()

CONJUNCTIVE COLOURING (fluoride) **ABSENT ()** LIGHT () MODERATE () SEVERE ()

CORNEAL COLOURING **ABSENT ()** LIGHT () MODERATE () GRAVE/CEP()

CORNEA/ TEAR SIGNS **ABSENT ()** MILD/DAMAGED MENISCUS () MODERATE () SEVERE ()

EYELIDS/GLDS.MEIBOMIUS DGM VARIABLE() DGM FREQUENT () TRIQ/SIMBL/QUERAT ()

TFBUT Variable () lower 10 () lower 5 () immediate ()

Schirmmer test I and II (Baseline and reflex) variable () lower 10 () lower 5 () lower 2 Other signs on examination CVA ODOE

Ectoscopy : exophthalmos () palp retraction () ectropion () lagophthalmos () entropion ()

Bio:

Eyelids: cir.palp() blepharitis() meibomitis() trichiasis() alveolar edge() AADL()

Conjunctiva: cir.conj () ptg/pinguecula () hyperaemia conj ()

Cornea: cir. Cornea () ptg () dellen () oedema () opacities ()

Cataract : s() n ()

Bio c fluoride/ rose bengal : normal meniscus () diminished meniscus () mucus () filaments () debris ()

Tonometry:

Fundoscopy: no RD () RDNP () RDP ()

RD staging: mild () moderate () severe ()

DEWS GRAU:

2* evaluation : 1 week after treatment

OSE symptoms neverf) infrequent () frequent () incapacitating ()

Visual symptoms neverf) infrequent () frequent () incapacitating ()

CONJUNCTIVAL INJECTION **ABSENT ()** MIGHTY () MODERATE () SEVERE ()

CONJUNCTIVE COLOURING (fluoride) **ABSENT ()** MIGHTY () MODERATE () SEVERE ()

CORNEAL COLOURING **ABSENT ()** LIGHT () MODERATE () SEVERE/CEP()

SIGNS CORNEA/ TEAR **ABSENT ()** MILD/DIM.MENISCUS () MODERATE () SEVERE () EYELIDS/GLDS.MEIBOMIUS DGM VARIABLE () DGM FREQUENT ()

TRIQ/SIMBL/QUERAT ()

Bio c fluoride/ rose bengal: normal meniscus () diminished meniscus () mucus () filaments () debris () **DEWS GRADE:**

evaluation : 2 weeks after treatment

OSE symptoms never() infrequent () frequent () disabling ()

Visual symptoms neverf) infrequent () frequent () incapacitating ()

CONJUNCTIVAL INJECTION **ABSENT ()** MILD () MODERATE () SEVERE ()

CONJUNCTIVE COLOURING (fluoride) **ABSENT ()** MILD () MODERATE () SEVERE ()

CORNEAL COLOUR **ABSENT ()** MILD () MODERATE () SEVERE/CEP()

SIGNS CONCERN/LAGRIMA **ABSENT ()** MIGHTY/DIMMED meniscus () MODERATE () SEVERE () PALLPEBRAS/GLDS.MEIBOMIUS DGM VARIABLE))

FREQUENT DGM () TRIQ/SIMBL/QUERAT () **Bio c fluoride/rose cane:** normal meniscus () reduced meniscus () mucus () filaments () debris ()

DEWS GRAU:

4? evaluation: 3 weeks after treatment

OSE symptoms never() infrequent () frequent () disabling ()

Visual symptoms neverf) infrequent () frequent () incapacitating ()

CONJUNCTIVAL INJECTION **ABSENT ()** MILD () MODERATE () SEVERE ()

CONJUNCTIVE COLOURING (fluoride) **ABSENT ()** MILD () MODERATE () SEVERE ()

CORNEAL COLOUR **ABSENT ()** MILD () MODERATE () SEVERE/CEP()

CORNEA/ TEAR SIGNS ABSENT () MILD/DAMAGED MENISCUS () MODERATE () SEVERE ()

EYELIDS/GLDS.MEIBOMIUS VARIABLE DGM)) FREQUENT DGM () TRIQ/SIMBL/QUERAT ()

Bio c fluoride/ rose bengal: normal meniscus () diminished meniscus () mucus () filaments () debris ()

DEWS GRAU:

5ª evaluation : 4 weeks after treatment

OSE symptoms neverí) infrequent () frequent () incapacitating ()

Visual symptoms never() infrequent () frequent () disabling ()

CONJUNCTIVAL INJECTION **ABSENT ()** MILD () MODERATE () SEVERE ()

CONJUNCTIVE COLOURING (fluoride) **ABSENT ()** MILD () MODERATE)) SEVERE))

CORNEAL COLOUR **ABSENT))** MILD)) MODERATE)) SEVERE /CEP))

CORNEA/ TEAR SIGNS **ABSENT))** MILD/DIM.MENISCUS)) MODERATE)) SEVERE))

EYELIDS/GLDS.MEIBOMIUS VARIABLE DGM)) FREQUENT DGM () TRIQ/SIMBL/QUERAT ()

Bio c fluoride/ rose bengal: normal meniscus () diminished meniscus () mucus () filaments () debris ()

DEWS GRADE

I authorise my data to be published or presented at any scientific event, provided my identity is preserved, contributing to research into dry eye in diabetic patients.

I also authorise the treatment necessary for my case, and this ophthalmological examination and anamnesis.

Knowing that I can give up on being included in the project at any time, and also that if I undergo treatment with platelet concentrate I won't have an anus.

Signature:

APPENDIX B - Informed Consent Form

Informed Consent Form

We invite the patient, ____ below identified, attended at the Cornea Sector of the Ophthalmology Service of the Dr Alberto Antunes University Hospital, in Maceió - AL, who declares that he/she has been informed that he/she is participating in the scientific research **entitled "The use of platelet concentrate in dry eye in diabetic patients". The** justification for the project is mainly due to morbidity, with a high risk of complications due to severe dry eye (chronic pain, corneal opacities, corneal ulcers, low vision), which occurs frequently in diabetic patients. The project will be approved by the Research Ethics Committee, which is an interdisciplinary and independent collegiate body that exists in institutions that carry out research involving human beings in Brazil, created to defend the interests of the subjects in their integrity and dignity and to contribute to the development of research within ethical standards (Norms and Regulatory Guidelines for Research Involving Human Beings). After approval by the Research Ethics Committee (Av. Lourival Melo Mota, s/n, Cidade Universitária - Maceió - AL, tel. (82) 32141069, opening hours Monday to Friday from 8am to 1.30pm) and CONEP (SEPN 510 Norte Bloco A, Brasília-DF, tel. (61) 3315587, opening hours from 8am to 8pm), the patient will first undergo anamnesis and routine ophthalmological examination to diagnose dry eye. The patient chosen to take part in the project will undergo venipuncture for blood collection at HEMOAL (Alagoas Haemocentre). Platelet apheresis will be carried out, and after blood cultures and serologies, platelet concentrate eye drops (POC) will be made and used to treat dry eye for 1 month and will be assessed weekly. The sample of biological material that is not used will be discarded. The main objective of this research is to determine the prevalence of dry eye in diabetic patients and to assess clinical improvement with the use of CCP in patients who are refractory to conventional treatment. The existing alternative treatment is lubricants in eye drops or gel, and the participant has already used this treatment and has been refractory to this usual therapy.

The participating patient will be informed that they can have all the information they want about the study, now or at any time and that the information will be provided by the research coordinator: Profa Eurica A N. Ribeiro who can be located at the Federal University of Alagoas - UFAL, located at Av. Lourival de Melo Mota s/n, Cidade Universitária, telephone (82)32141069, and by researcher Dr Marina Viegas Moura Rezende Ribeiro, an ophthalmologist and master's student at Ufal, located at Av.Lourival de Melo Mota s/n, Cidade Universitária, telephone (82)32141069.

The participant will be informed of the risk of an accident during blood collection, which may form a red stain on my arm, which will disappear within a few days without any major problems.

You will be informed that the risks of infection with the use of these eye drops are rare in the literature, since a haemoculture is carried out on your blood before preparing the eye drops, and they will be frozen at low temperatures. In addition, a prophylactic antibiotic eye drop will be used in conjunction with this treatment. However, if there is any type of eye infection, it will be treated immediately with specific antibiotic therapy and treatment with CCP will be suspended.

The patient will be informed that all information will be collected, protected and archived in a secure place by the researcher in charge, kept secret and that their name will not appear anywhere. That at any time they can refuse to take part in the research, or withdraw their consent, without any penalty or prejudice.

You will be informed that there **are no personal expenses** for you at any time during the study. **There is** also **no financial compensation** related to your participation. In the event of personal injury, direct or indirect, immediate or delayed, we guarantee the research participant legally established compensation and free treatment for as long as necessary. We will reimburse the patient and their companion, when necessary, for all expenses related to participation in the project, such as transport to and from appointments and meals on these dates.

By voluntarily agreeing to take part in this study, they authorise the researcher to use the results of these tests for research purposes, provided that their anonymity is guaranteed.

Declares to have understood and agreed to all the terms of this free and informed consent.

This form will be signed in two copies, one of which will remain with the researcher responsible and the other with the patient or their legal guardian. All pages must be initialled by the researcher responsible and the participant.

Maceió, 2014.

____
Signature
____
Coordinating Researcher
____
Collaborating Researcher
____
Co-supervisor

Collaborator

Collaborator

ANNEX A - Ethics committee approval

CONEP: 30435114.6.0000.5013

Trial Registration: Use of platelet-rich plasma in diabetic patients with dry eye disease

Institution: Brazilian Clinical Trials Registry (Rebec)

Registry number: RBR-96t463

URL (trial URL):http://www.ensaiosclinicos.gov.br/rg/RBR-96t463/

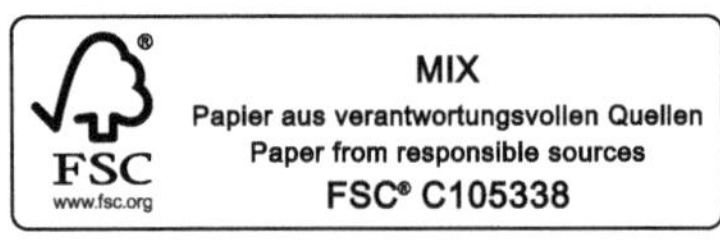

Printed by Books on Demand GmbH, Norderstedt / Germany